医学论文英文写作

English Medical Paper Writing

刘佳佳　著

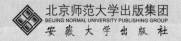

北京师范大学出版集团
BEIJING NORMAL UNIVERSITY PUBLISHING GROUP
安徽大学出版社

图书在版编目（CIP）数据

医学论文英文写作 / 刘佳佳著 . -- 合肥：安徽大学出版社，2024. 7.
--ISBN 978-7-5664-2824-0

Ⅰ. R

中国国家版本馆 CIP 数据核字第 2024830FM7 号

医 学 论 文 英 文 写 作
Yixue Lunwen Yingwen Xiezuo

刘佳佳　著

出版发行：北京师范大学出版集团
　　　　　安 徽 大 学 出 版 社
　　　　　（安徽省合肥市肥西路 3 号　邮编 230039）
　　　　　www.bnupg.com
　　　　　www.ahupress.com.cn
印　　刷：合肥华苑印刷包装有限公司
经　　销：全国新华书店
开　　本：710 mm × 1010 mm 1/16
印　　张：10.5
字　　数：217 千字
版　　次：2024 年 7 月第 1 版
印　　次：2024 年 7 月第 1 次印刷
定　　价：39.90 元
ISBN 978-7-5664-2824-0

策划编辑：李　雪　　　　　　　　装帧设计：李　雪　李　军
责任编辑：李　雪　　　　　　　　美术编辑：李　军
责任校对：高婷婷　　　　　　　　责任印制：陈　如　孟献辉

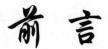 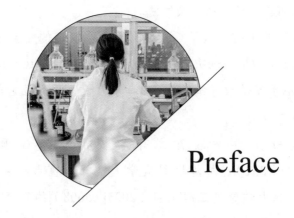

Preface

  国际医学期刊是世界各国医学研究人员传递和分享学术研究成果的重要载体。通过在国际期刊上发表论文，医学研究人员能够向医学界传递自己的研究成果和思想，为世界各国同行提供宝贵的参考和指导，推动学术交流和合作，促进医学领域的进步和发展。同时，在国际医学期刊发表高水平研究论文体现了研究人员的学术能力和贡献，有助于提高我国医学人才在国际上的影响力和竞争力。

  不了解国际期刊论文的写作规范和语言特征，就不可能用英语撰写和发表高质量的医学研究型论文。因此，医学研究人员需要一本总结论文英文写作规范的著作，引导他们从语篇布局、句法结构、词汇选择等语言层面更深入地了解国际医学期刊研究论文的写作范式，增加发表机会。本书旨在帮助读者掌握医学论文英文写作的技巧和规范，提升论文的质量和影响力。

  本书参照国际医学期刊研究论文的常见范式，以高级别国际医学期刊中近几年的研究论文为语料，分析论文的写作结构和语言特征。笔者按照常见写作结构和流程，将本书划分为概论、标题页、引言部分、方法部分、结果部分、讨论部分、文内引用、致谢与参考文献、摘要、投稿信函，共十章。本书还结合语言学理论，从语篇体裁、语步、句法、元话语等角度剖析、归纳语料中有参考意义的语言特征，为读者提供

"脚手架"，引导读者从宏观层面到微观层面逐步观察、分析、学习、模仿、掌握医学论文的英文写法。

本书基于国际医学期刊编辑委员会制定的《生物医学期刊投稿的统一要求》（*Uniform Requirements for Manuscripts Submitted to Biomedical Journals*）等学术写作规范，参考了大量医学及语言学权威文献，确保其学术性与权威性。

本书作为安徽省高等学校质量工程项目（2018mooc279，2019jyxm0252）、蚌埠医科大学人文社科重点项目（2023byzd147sk）、蚌埠医科大学质量工程项目（2023jyxm08）的研究成果，兼具理论性、学术性、实用性及新颖性，内容丰富、可读性强、可操作性强，希望读者能够通过阅读本书掌握用英语撰写医学期刊研究论文的技能，不断实践和思考，提升医学英语学术素养，提高论文的录用率和影响力，在医学研究领域取得更大的成就。

最后，我想对每位拿起这本书的读者说："愿您在医学论文英语写作的道路上不断进步，不仅作为一名写作者，更作为一名科学研究者和探索者。"

刘佳佳

2024 年 5 月

目 录

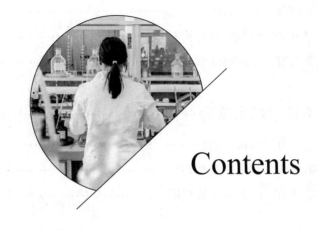

Contents

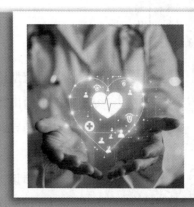

第一章
概　论

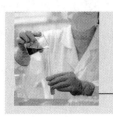

第一节 医学研究型论文的概念

医学研究型论文是以特定体裁和方式撰写及发表的，描述医学原创性研究成果的书面出版报告。医学研究型论文和综述论文等其他论文的不同之处在于它是问题导向性的，写作目的是解决某个医学领域尚未解决的问题或填补某项空白。

医学英语论文是医学工作者用英语撰写的，可能在以英语为母语或官方语言的国家的医学期刊或非英语国家英文版医学期刊上发表的医学论文。撰写并发表医学英语论文是为了更好地与国际同行交流自己的医学研究成果，同时让自己的研究成果在国际上得到认可。医学英语论文包括论著、研究型论文、文献综述、述评和病例报告等不同体裁，其格式与写作方法有所不同。

医学研究型英语论文往往呈现出一些特有的语言特征，包括医学术语的使用，学术名词、报告动词等词汇的使用，特定的时态、语态等语法特征，模糊语、增强语等元话语的使用，分阶语步的使用等文本和语言特征。

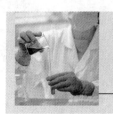

第二节 医学研究型论文的结构

医学研究型论文是医学界的科研成果交流工具。早期期刊发表的论文往往是冗长的描述性论文。20世纪以来，期刊开始要求稿件写作严谨、条理清晰。期刊版面比较稀缺，这就要求作者表述简洁。

用于投稿的医学研究型论文通常是由标题页（title page）、摘要（abstract）、关键词（key words）、正文（main text）、致谢（acknowledgements）和参考文献（references）构成的。其中正文通常包含引言（introduction）、方法（methods）、结果（results）和讨论（discussion）部分，此即所谓的IMRAD结构。这种格式可以清晰地呈现整个研究过程。

期刊编辑们认为IMRAD结构是交流研究成果最简单、最合理的方式，大大节省了期刊的空间，方便作者组织和撰写稿件，也方便编辑、审稿人和读者按结构索引、阅读论文。引言部分主要介绍作者为什么做这项工作，其目的是什么。方法部分介绍作者使用什么材料，以及是如何使用它们的。结果部分说明作者发现了什么。讨论部分阐述作者的发现意味着什么。

第二章
标题页

根据国际医学期刊编辑委员会（International Committee of Medical Journal Editors, ICMJE）制定的《生物医学期刊投稿的统一要求》，论文标题页主要包括：①论文标题（article title）；②作者姓名及所属机构（authors' names and institutional affiliations）；③研究工作的所属部门或单位名称（the name of the department[s] and institution[s] to which the work should be attributed）；④可能存在的放弃署名者（disclaimers, if any）；⑤通讯作者的联系信息（contact information for corresponding authors）；⑥资助、设备、药品来源（source[s] of support in the form of grants, equipment, drugs, or all of these）；⑦栏外标题（a running head）；⑧正文字数（word counts）；⑨图表数量（the number of figures and tables）。本章就医学期刊研究论文标题页中的论文标题、作者姓名及所属机构三大主要内容的英文写作进行详细说明。

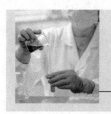

第一节
论文标题

论文标题是从研究论文中提炼出的精华部分，和摘要一样，虽然出现在文章的开始部分，但往往是在完成论文主体部分之后才确定的。论文标题的质量至关重要，因为作为一篇论文的第一部分，读者通常会通过标题去判断论文的内容是否和自己的研究相关。它可以吸引读者进一步阅读，或者让读者失去继续阅读的兴趣。

论文标题是用一定逻辑关系连接起来的短语或句子，它是论文内容的一面镜子，应遵循准确、简明、有吸引力三大基本原则，在能吸引读者关注并且准确概括研究的内容、范围及方法的前提下尽量把标题压缩到最短。

第一个原则"准确"，指英文标题应能够准确地反映研究的内容、范围及方法等重要信息，概括论文的重要论点。例如以下两个英文标题：

① Action of antibiotics on bacteria

（抗生素对细菌的作用）

② Inhibition of growth of *Mycobacterium tuberculosis* by streptomycin

（链霉素对结核分枝杆菌的抑制作用）

　　第一个标题很宽泛，既没有具体说明抗生素、细菌的种类，也没有说明到底是什么样的作用。而第二个标题相较于第一个而言，具体描述了抗生素的种类是 streptomycin（链霉素），细菌的种类是 *Mycobacterium tuberculosis*（结核分枝杆菌），并说明了链霉素对结核分枝杆菌所产生的是抑制作用（inhibition of growth）。因此第二个标题更为准确。

　　第二个原则"简明"，指英文标题要简练，长度要适当，在准确反映论文内容的前提下应尽量缩到最短。在不影响语义表达的前提下，尽量省略较为宽泛的词汇和短语。例如可以省略 a study of, an investigation into, a survey of, an analysis of, a comparison of 等，使标题更加简明，因为省略之后并不会影响读者理解题意。

　　第三个原则"有吸引力"，这需要作者在标题中涵盖文章的关键词信息，这样才能吸引读者关注，方便读者检索。

一、标题的常见形式和要素

　　医学研究型论文的英语标题通常有名词性标题、复合标题、陈述句标题、疑问句标题四种形式。

（一）名词性标题

　　名词性标题是医学研究型论文里常用的一种标题形式，它通常用来概括论文的主题，因此通常会包含论文中的关键词。名词性标题一般由名词短语或动名词短语构成。

　　名词短语式标题由一个以上的名词或名词短语加上修饰成分构成，它并不是一个完整的句子。书写这种标题时应该首先确定标题的中心词，然后再以正确的顺序进行修饰。例如标题"Long-term effects of hepatitis B immunization of infants in preventing liver cancer（婴儿乙肝免疫预防肝癌的长期效果）"是以名词性短语 long-term effects 为中心词，加上介词引导的多重后置定语"of hepatitis B immunization of infants in preventing liver cancer"构成的。

动名词短语式标题是动名词引导的短语式标题，也不是一个完整句。例如，标题"Locating ambulatory medical care facilities for the elderly（为老年人设立流动医疗设施）"是动名词 locating 引导的动名词短语式标题。

（二）复合标题

复合标题在医学研究型论文中也很常见，通常由两个连续的短语构成，第一个短语为论文的主标题，第二个短语为副标题，主、副标题之间一般用冒号连接。论文的副标题一般用于进一步限定主标题或对主标题进行补充说明，例如标题"Anxiety and cardiovascular symptoms: The modulating role of insomnia（焦虑与心血管症状：失眠的调节作用）"的副标题强调了研究重点，再比如标题"Effect of nonoxynol-9 gel on urogenital gonorrhea and chlamydial infection: A randomized controlled trial（壬苯醇醚 -9 凝胶对泌尿生殖道淋病和衣原体感染的作用：一项随机对照试验）"的副标题解释了研究方法。

另外，有的复合标题以问句作为副标题，提出研究问题，这种方式更能吸引读者的注意。例如标题"Growth hormone: A new therapy for heart failure?（生长激素能否成为心衰的一种新疗法？）"就是一个"短语＋问句"形式的复合标题。

（三）陈述句标题

医学研究型论文中偶尔会出现由一个完整的陈述句作为论文标题的情况。这种标题一般偏长，语义完整，便于读者理解。需要注意的是，陈述句标题的句尾一般不需要加句号。例如标题"Dietary cholesterol is carcinogenic for human colon cancer（膳食胆固醇是人类结肠癌的致癌物）"就是一个陈述句标题。

（四）疑问句标题

以疑问句作为医学研究型论文标题的情况同样不常见。疑问句使得标题具有探讨性的语气，容易引发读者的阅读兴趣。疑问句标题后需要加问号，例如标题"Does the chronic fatigue syndrome involve the autonomic nervous system?（慢性疲劳综合征会累及自主神经系统么？）"就是一个疑问句标题。

二、标题的常见语言规范

作者用英语撰写医学研究型论文时，应参考不同医学期刊的具体要求，通常此类论文标题遵循以下语言规范。

（一）尽量避免使用缩略语

标题中应尽可能少用或者不用缩略语。如果一定要用，就尽量使用读者熟知的、已经得到行业认可的常用缩略语。例如标题"Research on the relationship between human sperm DNA integrity and sperm parameters in male infertility（不育症患者精子 DNA 完整性与精液相关参数的研究）"中使用的缩略语 DNA 要比其所代表的全称 deoxyribonucleic acid（脱氧核糖核酸）更为读者所熟知。再比如表示获得性免疫缺陷综合征（acquired immunodeficiency syndrome）的缩略语 AIDS，表示核磁共振成像（unclear magnetic resonance imaging）的缩略语 NMRI，也是可以在标题中使用的缩略语。

（二）尽量避免使用数字

标题中应尽量避免使用数字，例如标题"Physical and chemical studies of human blood serum: A study of 2158 cases of nephritis（人类血清的理化研究：2158 例肾炎的研究）"中并不需要精确地说明样本量，可以使用 large-scale study 来描述研究的规模。

（三）标题中的大小写

医学期刊对论文中英语标题的大小写要求不尽相同，需要作者在投稿前按照各期刊的要求书写英语标题。但常见的书写形式主要有两种。

第一种形式：标题中每个实词和 4 个字母及以上的虚词的首字母大写。实词指除介词、冠词和连词等虚词以外的有实际含义的词。例如标题"A Successful Operation on a Pair of Female Twins With Conjoined Liver（一例腹部连体共肝女性双胞胎成功分离手术）"中，除了题首的不定冠词 a 要大写，标题中的不定冠词 a、介词 on、of 都为小写。而由 4 个字母组成的介词 with 采用了首字母大写的形式。

第二种形式：要求标题第一个词的首字母大写，其余字母小写。但专有名词或通用缩略语中应该大写的字母仍然要大写。例如在标题"Differential diagnoses of uterine leiomyomas and leiomyosarcomas using DNA and RNA sequencing（应用 DNA 和 RNA 测序对子宫肌瘤和平滑肌肉瘤进行鉴别诊断）"中，除了第一个单词 differential 的首字母、通用缩略语 DNA 和 RNA 使用了大写，其余字母都采用了小写。

另外，如果是复合标题，副标题第一个单词的首字母通常也要大写。例如标题"Renal hypertension: A clinical analysis of 655 cases（655 例肾性高血压临床分析）"中，主标题和副标题的第一个单词的首字母 Renal 和不定冠词 A 都使用了大写。

（四）标题中的冠词

近些年，医学论文英语标题中的冠词使用有简化的趋势，在不影响表达的前提下，冠词均可省略。标题起始处的定冠词一般要省略。例如标题"CT perfusion imaging in preoperative grading of astrocytoma（CT 灌注成像在星形细胞瘤术前分级中的应用）"。标题起始处的不定冠词一般要保留。例如标题"A prospective natural-history study of coronary atherosclerosis（冠状动脉粥样硬化的前瞻性自然史研究）"。

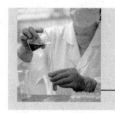

第二节
作者姓名

一、作者身份的界定

国际医学期刊编辑委员会在《生物医学期刊投稿的统一要求》中规定，作者身份的确定必须符合以下三条标准：①对概念和设计、数据获取或数据分析和解释有重大贡献；②撰写论文或对其中重要内容作重大修改；③同意最终稿的发表。论文的所有署名作者都必须具备以上三个条件，仅仅筹集资金、收集数据或对研究小组进行一般性的管理是不足以成为作者的。所有具有署名资格的人都应被列为作者。

二、作者英文署名特点

作者署名一般位于论文标题的正下方，按照作者的贡献大小依次排列。除此之外，署名的时候还要注意以下几个方面。

首先，国外作者姓名的首字母要大写，作者姓名中如果含有中间名的首字母，需要将其大写，书写在姓名中间，并在后面加上英文句点。例如Daniel E. Spratt。

中国作者英文署名要以汉语拼音的形式书写。一般来说其姓和名拼音的首字母要大写，采用名写在前、姓写在后的方式，复名直接连写或用连字符连接。例如以下屠呦呦团队在国际权威医学期刊《新英格兰医学杂志》上发表的有关"青蒿素抗药性"的文章中，屠呦呦、王继刚等作者的署名都遵循了名前姓后的原则，名和姓之间空一格，复名直接连写：

A Temporizing Solution to "Artemisinin Resistance"

Jigang Wang, Ph.D., Chengchao Xu, Ph.D., Fulong Liao, B.S., Tingliang Jiang,

M.S., Sanjeev Krishna, Sc.D., and Youyou Tu, B.S.

如果一篇论文有多个作者，作者姓名间要以逗号分隔。通常情况下，作者姓名的右上角会标注阿拉伯数字（1, 2, 3⋯⋯）或小写字母 (a, b, c⋯⋯) 以表示不同的作者单位，标注星号（*）代表通讯作者（corresponding author）身份。

有的期刊要求作者署名时，在姓名的后面附上作者的最高学位。如上例中，Ph.D.（Doctor of Philosophy）表示博士学位，B.S.（Bachelor of Science）表示理学学士，M.S.（Master of Science）表示理学硕士，Sc.D.（Doctor of Science）表示理学博士。再比如M.B.（Bachelor of Medicine）表示医学学士，M.M.（Master of Medicine）表示医学硕士，M.D.（Doctor of Medicine）表示医学博士。

投稿时需参考期刊的具体署名要求。另外，建议作者尽量采用相对固定的英文姓名表达形式，以减少在文献检索和论文引用中被他人误解的可能性。

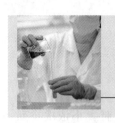

在作者署名之后，通常还要附上作者的工作单位信息。工作单位信息一般包含作者所属工作机构及其所在地等信息。根据不同期刊的要求，这部分内容通常书写于作者署名的下一行，也有的期刊要求写在摘要旁边或文末的附录（appendix）中，目前很多国际医学期刊要求将单位名称写在论文首页下方的脚注中。

用英文表述工作单位时，需要按由小到大的顺序表示各级别，如"课题组/研究组→科室/部门→医院/研究所/校名→市→省/州→国家"。完整书写单位名称，每个实词的首字母大写，避免使用单位名称的缩写形式。例如 Artemisinin Research Center and the Institute of Chinese Materia Medica, China Academy of Chinese Medical Sciences, Beijing, China，各级别之间以逗号相隔。

论文标题页中除了标题和作者信息两大部分，标题页中可能还会涉及 Running head（栏外标题）、Correspondence（通讯作者的联系信息）、Sponsorship（资助来源）、Word count（正文字数）及 Number of figures and tables（图表数量）等其他信息。各个期刊都有其特定的书写形式，投稿时要参照要求进行书写。

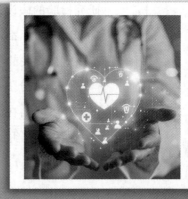

第三章
引言部分

论文正文部分位于摘要及关键词部分之后，通常以 IMRAD 的格式呈现，也就是 introduction，methods，results 和 discussion 四个部分。本章将探讨如何书写医学研究型论文正文中的第一个部分"引言"。

《生物医学期刊投稿的统一要求》对引言部分的内容进行了说明，"引言为研究提供背景（即问题的性质及其意义）。说明该研究的目的，或是经该研究检验的假设；当以问题的形式陈述时，研究目标往往更加明确。主要目标和次要目标都应该是清晰明确的，应该描述任何预先设定的亚组分析。只提供直接相关的参考文献，不包括正在报告的工作的数据或结论"。

引言部分的主要作用是介绍研究背景、提出研究问题以及阐明研究目的。作者要站在读者的角度，设法吸引读者的阅读兴趣，简洁精炼地介绍论文中所做的研究，逐步引导其了解该研究。

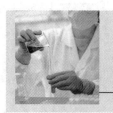

第一节 结构和语步

Swales（1990）提出了体裁分析（genre analysis）中的修辞语步（rhetorical moves），用于研究论文的修辞组织模式（表3-1）。它的功能是描述文本的交际目的，根据交际目的或修辞语步对文本中的各种话语单元进行分类。因此，语步指的是文本中某一部分的特定交际功能。每一个语步都有自己的目的，又与文本的整体交际目的相辅相成。这些语步的目的决定了文本交流的基本原理，而该基本原理又决定了话语的图式结构，影响并制约着文本内容和风格的选择。

表 3-1　研究论文引言部分的语步结构模型

语步 1（M1）：确立研究领域（establishing a territory）

　　步骤 1（S1）：建立中心主题（claiming centrality）（可选）

　　步骤 2（S2）：概括主题内容（making topic generalization[s]）（可选）

　　步骤 3（S3）：综述前人研究（reviewing previous research）（必选）

语步 2（M2）：确立研究地位（establishing a niche）

　　步骤 1（S1）：反面论证（counter claiming）（可选）

　　步骤 2（S2）：指出研究不足（indicating a gap）（可选）

　　步骤 3（S3）：提出研究问题（question raising）（必选）

语步 3（M3）：占领研究地位（occupying the niche）

　　步骤 1（S1）：提出研究目的（stating objectives）（必选）

　　步骤 2（S2）：宣布当前研究（announcing present research）（可选）

　　步骤 3（S3）：宣布主要结果（announcing principal findings）（可选）

　　步骤 4（S4）：介绍文章结构（indicating article structure）（可选）

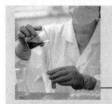

**第二节
建立中心主题、概括主题内容**

一、写作内容及特点

　　建立中心主题、概括主题内容是确立研究领域中的重要一环，作者需要通过介绍论文研究主题的相关背景及重要性向读者阐述该领域的现状和问题，以及研究这一主题的意义。

表 3-2 引言样例

Acceleration of BMI in Early Childhood and Risk of Sustained Obesity

The overall prevalence of childhood obesity remains very high, and the prevalence of very high levels of body-mass index (BMI) for age in children is still rising. Most adolescents who are obese remain so in adulthood. The early onset of obesity is associated with the emergence of related complications, including metabolic and cardiovascular disorders, even in childhood, and may lead to an increased risk of death in adulthood.

Ascertainment of the age at which obesity develops and determination of whether there are specific critical periods in childhood and adolescence that are characterized by accelerated and sustained weight gain are thus important and may aid in the development of effective preventive strategies.

Studies to predict the development of obesity on the basis of childhood BMI have suggested a positive correlation, but most have evaluated outcomes at a young age[1,2] or have had a relatively late baseline evaluation,[3] a short observation period,[4,5] or a small sample size.[6-9] The exact pattern of weight gain during childhood that leads to sustained obesity is unclear and warrants longitudinal data that cover the entire age span from infancy to adolescence in a population of an appropriate sample size.

In the current study, we tracked BMI in individual children from infancy to adolescence in a large population to determine the age at which children are most vulnerable to excessive weight gain that ultimately results in obesity in adolescence.

　　表 3-2 引言样例的第 1 段第 1 句中陈述了儿童肥胖的总体患病率一直很高，儿童中高体重指数的发生率持续上升的现状："The overall prevalence of childhood obesity remains very high, and the prevalence of very high levels of body-mass index (BMI) for age in children is still rising." 第 2、3 句指出了问题的严重性：早期肥胖可能会导致成年期的肥胖 "Most adolescents who are obese remain so in adulthood"，引发其他并发症 "associated with the emergence of related complications"，增加死亡的风险 "may lead to an increased risk of death in adulthood"，从而介绍了与论文标题《儿童早期体重指数的增加和持续肥胖的风险》这一主题相关的背景信息，建立了中心主题。

　　这篇引言的第二段概括了第一段中所提到的主题内容，强调了确定肥胖形成的年龄 "Most adolescents who are obese remain so in adulthood" 和确定儿童期和青春期是否存在以体重加速及持续增长为特征的特定关键时期 "determination of whether there are specific critical periods in childhood and adolescence that are characterized by accelerated and sustained weight gain" 两个因素在制定预防肥胖的有效策略时的重要性。

在这一部分作者还可能需要对主题相关的概念或关键性术语进行解释，并在首次出现的完整术语后加括号标注其缩略词。一旦缩略词被引入，在后续的论文部分中就应使用缩略词，例如表 3-2 引言第一段中引入了"身体质量指数（body-mass index）"的缩略词 BMI，后面再次出现该概念时就应直接使用。

二、常用语法和句型

在介绍研究背景时，通常使用一般现在时，表示已被接受或确定的事实。研究型论文通常以公认或已确立的事实开头，这可以确保读者与作者共享相同级别的背景信息，做好阅读文章的准备，例如，"It is widely known that..."。而在表示背景或趋势对该领域造成的影响时多用现在完成时，例如，"Over the last few years, many studies have been focused on..."。

建立中心主题、概括主题内容这一语步通常会使用以下表示背景、趋势或重要性的信号词（signal words）（表 3-3）。

表 3-3　表示背景、趋势或重要性的信号词

challenging	significant	recent
major	vital	possible
common	important	nowadays
considerable	potential	beneficial
current	central	advantage
essential	popular	well-known
increasing	rapid	widespread
leading	typical	concern

这一语步的常用句型有：

① 表示趋势或影响。

The prevalence of...is increasing at an alarming rate in...

...is a growing public health concern worldwide.

The past…have seen an increasing…in…

The number of…grows at a fast pace.

…has received considerable attention.

…is a common condition which has considerable impact on…

With the medical advance in…, …has generated considerable interest.

It is generally accepted that…

It is well established that… can impair…

…is associated with increased risk of…

…is one of the most widely used…

② 表示重要性。

There is evidence that…plays a crucial role in…

…has contributed significantly to…

…plays a/an key/vital/crucial/essential/important/significant/fundamental role in ensuring/reducing/preventing the treatment of/the regulation of/ protecting against/the maintenance of/the pathogenesis of…

…has been shown to be essential for…

…has long been recognized as one of the key…

The importance of…has been demonstrated by…

…is fundamental to…

Evidence suggests that… is among the most important factors for…

③ 定义、描述术语或概念。

…is a common disorder characterized by…

…can be referred to as…

…can be defined as…

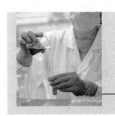

第三节
综述前人研究、指出研究不足

一、写作内容及特点

在总结了研究背景，强调了研究主题的重要性之后，作者通常需要进行文献综述，系统回顾国内外最新的相关研究。文献综述可以让读者了解本研究主题的最新成果和动态，以及本研究所依据的信息来源。作者通过文献综述对前人的研究表示尊敬，这也能让编辑和审稿人看到作者做了充分的研究准备工作。文献综述部分一般属于引言部分（也有些期刊要求将其单独设置为一个部分），通常较为简短（1~2段），没有必要引用多篇描述同一现象的论文，更重要的是总结前人成果、为读者提供相关领域研究的综合性概述和客观评价。文献综述一般包括两个步骤：综述前人研究（具体提及或总结相关的工作），和指出其研究中的不足（评论其中的问题、局限性、错误或空白）。

第一个步骤"综述前人研究"是对前人（包括自己）工作的引用，包括实际引用（通常伴随着对特定研究人员姓名的引用），如"斯韦尔斯等人报告说……（Swales et al. reported that...）"，或对前人研究的一般性引用，如"研究人员已经证明……（Researchers have shown that...）"。综述文献时应按照一定的逻辑顺序，一般是时间顺序（文献出版顺序）或主题顺序（比如按不同研究方法、研究对象或研究理论的顺序组织文献）。

第二个步骤"指出研究中的不足"是指在综述了前人研究之后提出其中存在的不足之处，如"然而，斯韦尔斯等人未能发现任何……的病例（However, Swales et al. failed to identify any cases in which...）"，或前人尚未解决的问题，从而引出本论文的研究问题，或者提到了我们现有知识中仍然存在的空白，如"然而，我们仍然不知道……（However, ...is not known）"。上述两个例句的开头都是 However，它和其他对比连词（如 but, yet, although, in spite of, in contrast to 等）经常用来强化作者介绍当前研究的理由。但是在指出他人工作的局限性时，要尽量谨慎，通过间接、对抗性较弱的方式描述研究成果而不是研究人员的不足，比如可以用"The study of... did not identify..."（该研究并未证明……）代替"...failed to identify..."（该研究不能证明……）。

表 3-2 引言样例的第三段中作者回顾了前人基于儿童体重指数预测肥胖发展所做的相关研究，并指出了其中的缺陷：第 1 条和第 2 条参考文献的研究缺陷是在年龄较小时评估的结果（evaluated outcomes at a young age），第 3 条是基线评估相对较晚（a relatively late baseline evaluation），第 4 条和第 5 条是观察期较短（a short observation period），而第 6 条到第 9 条是样本量较小（a small sample size）。

这一段还指出了前人尚未研究、解决的问题：儿童期体重增加导致持续肥胖的确切模式（The exact pattern of weight gain during childhood that leads to sustained obesity is unclear），并且需要在适当样本量的人群中覆盖从婴儿期到青春期的整个年龄跨度的纵向数据（warrants longitudinal data that cover the entire age span from infancy to adolescence in a population of an appropriate sample size）。

作者在综述文献时，一般不会逐条地罗列相关文献中的研究，而是会在充分阅读了解各条文献中的研究之后，发现不同研究间的关联，找到一定的角度将它们进行多源整合（synthesizing），用自己的语言总结描述，从而为阐述本研究提供支撑。

比如下页这段文献综述样例中（表 3-4），作者对多条相关文献进行了多源整合。首先，作者以一个引导句（leading sentence）开始导入，表示已有研究表明在一些手术前进行抗生素预防可以减少术后感染的风险。在第二句中，作者综述了文献 7，这篇文献通过 19 个随机对照实验，表明预防性抗生素可以减少引产手术所引起的盆腔感染。而第三句表明作者经过了文献综述，发现目前还缺乏证据证明预防性抗生素对于流产手术的有效性，只有四项较小的单中心研究（第 4、9、10、11 条文献）表明预防性抗生素对于流产手术没有显著效果。在这一句中作者使用了 However 表示语义上的转折，说明作者发现了前人尚未研究或很少研究的问题（research gap）。在第四句中，作者又进一步指出了第三句中提到的四项研究中研究方法上的缺陷（methodological limitations），分别是研究规模小（small size）、抗生素剂量不足（inadequate antibiotic dose）、对研究方案的依从性差（poor adherence to the study protocol），从而为作者进行进一步的研究做铺垫。

表 3-4　文献综述样例

Antibiotic prophylaxis before some operations has been shown to reduce the risk of postoperative infections. A Cochrane review of 19 randomized, controlled trials of the use of antibiotic prophylaxis before uterine evacuation for induced termination of pregnancy showed that prophylactic antibiotics reduced pelvic infection for this specific indication.[7] However, for miscarriage surgery, evidence is lacking to show effectiveness, with four small, single-center studies showing no significant benefit from prophylactic antibiotics. In addition to small size,[4,9-11] these studies had other methodological limitations, including inadequate antibiotic dose[9] and poor adherence to the study protocol.[4]

二、常用语法和句型

通过下面的例句，我们可以观察到作者在综述前人研究具体内容时（他们做了什么）通常使用一般过去时（例 1），而在总结概括前人研究的特点时（他们如何总结评价该研究领域或自己的研究）通常使用现在完成时（例 2）。

例 1：

Previously, we provided the first evidence in humans that universal hepatitis B immunization in infancy can effectively reduce the incidence of liver cancer in children and adolescents.

此前，我们首次证明了人类在婴儿时期普及乙肝免疫可有效降低儿童期和青少年期的肝癌发病率。

例 2：

However, observational studies have shown that the administration of dopamine may be associated with rates of death that are higher than those associated with the administration of norepinephrine.

然而，观察性研究表明，使用多巴胺的死亡率可能高于使用去甲肾上腺素的死亡率。

通过下面两个例子我们可以发现作者基于文献综述指出前人研究的问题和不足之处，或陈述前人研究空白时往往会根据情况使用两种时态：①当使用 not certain、not clear、not known、remain unclear、unconvincing、questionable 等表示研究状态时，通常使用一般现在时（例3）；②当使用 conduct、pay、attention、to、focus、do、investigate 等研究性动词表示动作时，通常使用现在完成时（例4）。

例3：

Thus, dopamine and norepinephrine may have different effects on the kidney, but the clinical implications of these differences are still uncertain.

因此，多巴胺和去甲肾上腺素可能对肾脏有不同的影响，但这些影响差异的临床意义仍不确定。

例4：

However, few studies have investigated the clinical implications of their different effects of dopamine and norepinephrine on the kidney.

然而，很少有研究调查多巴胺和去甲肾上腺素对肾脏的不同作用所产生的临床意义。

用来综述前人研究、指出研究不足这一语步时通常会使用以下信号词（表3-5）。

表3-5　综述前人研究、指出研究不足的常用信号词

综述前人研究		指出研究不足	
analyzed	illustrated	inadequate	unclear
applied	improved	inconsistent	misleading
attempted	investigated	defect	not addressed
compared	measured	flaw	not studied
conducted	observed	gap	unsatisfactory
demonstrated	performed	lack	be confined to
described	predicted	limitation	demand clarification
designed	provided	problem	fail to
detected	reported	ineffective	need re-examination
developed	reviewed	insufficient	neglect
discovered	showed	of little value	overlook
established	studied	questionable	remain unknown

(continued)

综述前人研究		指出研究不足	
evaluated	tested	restricted	however
explored	used	uncertain	require clarification
found			

用来综述文献、指出研究不足常用的句型有：

① 综述文献。

Recent (previous/several) studies have suggested (shown/reported/demonstrated) that…

A large and growing body of literature has investigated…

Much of the literature since…emphasizes…

Over the past decade, most research in…has focused on…

There are a number of…studies which demonstrate…

A recent study by…found/reported that…

…et al. conducted/performed/carried out…in which…

It has been shown/observed/suggested/established/demonstrated that…

② 指出前人研究中的问题和缺陷。

Previous studies have failed to consider…

Previous studies have mostly/generally/typically/predominantly ignored…

Previous published studies on the effect of … are not consistent.

Prior research has been limited/restricted to/focused on…

To date, there has been little experimental/empirical evidence that…

Most of these studies have suffered from…

(small sample sizes/multiple design flaws/serious sampling problems/notable methodological weaknesses…)

③ 指出前人尚未研究的问题。

(Very) few studies have explored…/focused on…/measured…in humans/been conducted to determine the effect of…

However, few studies have explored…

So far, there has been little research on…

It is unclear/unknown whether…

Further studies on…are still necessary.

No study to date has investigated…

However, what is not yet clear/ known/ understood is…

Up to now, little research has been carried out on…

Further studies on…are still necessary/essential.

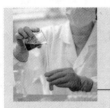

第四节
提出研究目的、问题或假设

一、写作内容及特点

引言部分的第三个语步是提出研究目的、问题或假设，指作者在分析前人研究中存在的问题或不足之处后，引出本研究的目的、将要解决的问题或要验证的假设。

提出研究目的这一步可以通过非常直接的陈述来完成，例如"本研究的目的是调查研究……（The objective of the study was to investigate… ）"；但有时候也可以采取更谨慎的方式，逐步过渡，比如添加 to address the problem, to fill in the gap 等过渡语将目的部分和前面两个语步自然连接在一起；另外，还可以通过简要提及研究方法或选择该研究方法的理由，例如"使用了……方法，目的是检验……（A/an…method was used to examine… ）"。通常在医学研究型论文的讨论部分会再次提及研究目的，与引言部分的研究目的相呼应。

表3-2引言样例的第四段中，作者引出了本论文中所进行的研究："In the current study, we tracked BMI in individual children from infancy to adolescence in a large population…（在此项研究中，我们追踪了大量人群从婴儿期到青

春期的体重指数……）"，并阐述了本研究的目的 "…to determine the age at which children are most vulnerable to excessive weight gain that ultimately results in obesity in adolescence（确定儿童在什么年龄最容易过度增重，从而最终导致青春期肥胖）"。

研究目标可以通过研究问题或研究假设进一步具体表达，从而让读者能更清晰、更有针对性地把握后面的内容，也更方便编辑和审稿人审核检验研究方法和结果是否一一对应地解决了研究问题、达到了研究目的。例如：Is Drug A an effective treatment for Disease B?

研究假设和研究问题一样，也能使研究目的更加具体。研究假设是对研究结果的预测，是在尚未得到验证的情况下回答研究问题。但研究假设并不是没有根据的任意猜测，而是基于现有的知识和理论。研究团队通过科学地设计研究方法和实验，验证假设是否成立。在学术研究中，假设常以相关性或效应来表达，作者通常直接陈述变量之间的预测关系。如果研究涉及统计假设检验，作者需要进行零假设（H0: null hypothesis）或备择假设（H1: alternative hypothesis）。零假设指变量之间没有关联的假设，例如对于上一段中提到的研究问题可以设定 Drug A will not significantly reduce symptoms associated with Disease B 这样的零假设；备择假设指变量之间有关联的假设，例如对于上一段中提到的研究问题可以有 Drug A will significantly reduce symptoms associated with Disease B 这样的备择假设。

二、常用语法和句型

相较于撰写论文的时间，作者进行研究的时间已经过去，因此通常使用一般过去时陈述本研究的目的，提出研究问题或假设。

提出研究目的、问题或假设这一语步通常会使用以下信号词（表 3-6）。

表 3-6 提出研究目的、问题或假设的信号词

aim	to compare	study
goal	to describe	project
purpose	to evaluate	test
objective	to facilitate	approach
	to improve	case

(continued)

to predict	innovation
to present	surgery
to demonstrate	therapy
to perform	medication
to investigate	disease
to examine	method
to design	
to report	

We... *v.* ed...

用来综述文献、指出研究不足的常用句型有：

① 阐述本研究的目的。

This study aimed to…

This study was designed to…

The aim/purpose/ objective of this study was to predict /establish /

determine /examine /compare /explore /identify …

The present study was designed with the objective of…

In order to investigate…, we…

In the present study we performed…

② 提出研究问题或假设。

Our research questions were…

The research questions in this study focused on…

This study aimed to address the following research questions: …

Another question is whether…

The key research question of this study was whether or not…

The following questions will be addressed:…

The hypothesis that will be tested is that…

　　大多数医学研究型论文作者都可以遵循以上几个语步撰写引言部分，为文章的第二大部分，即方法部分奠定基础。这并不是要求所有医学研究型论文的引文部分都按照以上步骤和内容书写，作者在论文写作过程中可以根据需要进行调整。

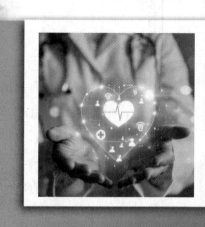

第四章
方法部分

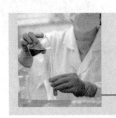

本章将探讨如何书写医学研究型论文正文中的第二部分"方法"。论文中常用 Methods 作为这一部分的标题，也有的论文会用 Methods and materials（方法与材料）。方法部分应包括研究计划或方案。

方法部分对于整篇论文来说具有重要的作用，它可以：①向读者提供有关研究步骤及所使用材料的详细信息，以便于其他研究人员复制实验；②证明研究结果的信度和效度。因此，作者在研究和写作过程中应该尽量借助学术领域内已被认可的研究方法和技术，引用领域内有重大影响和意义的研究或指导方针，给出研究过程中选择特定方法和步骤的理由。

Cotos et al. (2017) 基于大量研究论文提出了方法部分语步模型（表4-1）。其中第一语步是对方法部分的总体介绍；第二语步构成了方法部分的主体，提供有关方法步骤的细节信息；第三语步主要体现研究团队为了确保分析结果的可信度在处理分析数据过程中的严谨性。

表 4-1　方法部分语步模型（Cotos et.al., 2017）

语步 1（M1）：情境化研究方法（contextualizing study methods）

步骤 1（S1）：重述研究目标（recapturing the research purposes）

步骤 2（S2）：公布所使用的研究方法（announcing the method used）

步骤 3（S3）：将方法与该领域遵循的传统相联系（connecting methods to the traditions followed in the field）

步骤 4（S4）：描述环境（describing the setting）

步骤 5（S5）：描述主题（describing the subjects）

步骤 6（S6）：解释步骤 1~5（justifying S1~S5）

语步 2（M2）：描述研究（describing the study）

步骤 1（S1）：报告数据的获取方式或地点（reporting how or where the data were acquired）

步骤 2（S2）：描述数据特征（characterizing data）

步骤 3（S3）：描述实验 / 研究程序（describing experimental/study procedures）

步骤 4（S4）：命名和描述用于测试或进行其他任务的工具（naming and describing tools used to perform tests or other tasks）

步骤 5（S5）：描述实验所测试的变量或进行实验的条件（describing the variables being tested or conditions in which experiments were carried out）

步骤 6（S6）：解释步骤 1~5（justifying S1~S5）

语步 3（M3）：建立研究的可信度（establishing credibility of study）

步骤 1（S1）：准备数据（preparing the data）

步骤 2（S2）：操作数据（manipulating the data）

步骤 3（S3）：公布并描述统计工具和统计程序（announcing and describing the statistical tools and procedures）

步骤 4（S4）：说明所使用的统计规范（stating the statistical norms used）

步骤 5（S5）：解释步骤 1~2（justifying S1~S2）

在方法部分中，作者要围绕论文的研究问题，简洁、准确、清晰地描述和解释研究过程。通过方法部分语步模型，我们可以发现，作者在撰写该部分时，具体步骤遵循特定的模式，是一个从情境化研究方法到描述研究再到建立研究可信度的过程，是逐步告诉读者，作者是如何解决研究问题的过程。

方法部分往往会通过设置一些二级标题，系统化、分模块地阐述以上语步，使整体结构更清晰，也更易于理解。方法部分中常见的二级标题有 Study design（研究设计）、Study subjects（研究对象）、Outcome measures（结果测定方法）、Interventions（干预措施）、Data collection（数据收集）、Statistical analysis（统计学分析）等。此外，在设置二级标题时，我们还需要考虑研究类型、研究步骤、研究内容及期刊要求等因素。

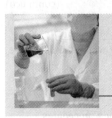

第二节
研究设计

很多医学研究型论文，尤其是临床研究论文的方法部分中会包含研究设计部分，也有的论文中没有单独设置研究设计部分，而是放在研究对象、测定方法等部分中进行介绍。这一部分简要介绍研究的大致情况，是方法部分第一语步"情境化研究方法"的描述，内容通常包含重述研究目标、公布所使用的研究方法及描述研究环境等。医学研究中常见的研究方法有prospective study（前瞻性研究）、retrospective study（回顾性研究）、crossover study（交叉研究）、single-blind study（单盲研究）、double-blind study（双盲研究）、controlled study（对照研究）、randomized study（随机研究）、experimental study（实验研究）等。描述研究环境一般包括对研究时间和地点（time and location）的描述。

例如，在表4-2里所描述的这一段研究设计样例中，作者简要介绍了研究方法"randomized, controlled, open-label study"，说明这是一项开放性、随机、对照的研究；描述了研究环境"Children's Hospital of Philadelphia... and University of Iowa""were reviewed and approved by The Committees for the Protection of Human Subjects"，说明这项研究分别是在美国的费城儿童医院及爱荷华大学进行的，该研究通过了这两个研究单位的人类受试者保护委员会的审查和批准，已获得相关研究资质。

我们看到，样例中的两个句子都使用了一般过去时的被动语态。

表 4-2　研究设计样例

> This randomized, controlled, open-label, phase 3 study was done with five surgeons at two sites in the USA (Children's Hospital of Philadelphia, Philadelphia, PA, and University of Iowa, Iowa City, IA). The study protocol and individual institutional informed consent documents were reviewed and approved by The Committees for the Protection of Human Subjects at Children's Hospital of Philadelphia and The University of Iowa Carver School of Medicine.

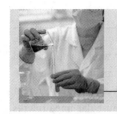

研究对象在英文论文中除了用 study subjects 表达，根据研究对象的不同，常用的二级标题还有 Participants、Study population、Study cohorts、Patients、Experimental animals 和 Cell culture 等。这一部分介绍了研究对象的大致情况，是对方法部分第二语步"描述研究"的阐述，内容通常包括报告数据的获取方式或地点和描述数据特征这两个步骤。医学研究对象的类型通常包括 patients（患者）、laboratory animals（实验室动物）、cells（细胞）、tissues（组织）等。

在书写研究对象部分时，作者应该清楚地描述研究对象的选择及排除标准（inclusion and exclusion criteria），例如表 4-3 的样例中，首先描述了研究对象的选择标准：65 years of age or older（65 岁以上），obese（肥胖），sedentary（久坐，每周的常规锻炼少于 1 小时），had a stable body weight and stable medication use for 6 months before enrollment（入组前体重稳定、用药稳定长达 6 个月）。

除了选择标准，作者还描述了研究对象的排除标准：persons who had severe cardiopulmonary disease（患有严重心肺疾病的人），who had musculoskeletal or neuromuscular impairments（有肌肉骨骼或神经肌肉损伤的人），who had cognitive impairments（有认知障碍的人），或者 who used drugs that affect bone metabolism（使用影响骨代谢药物的患者）。

我们可以发现，这一段中除了在描述研究对象加入研究组之前的体重和用药状况 "…had had a stable body weight (loss or gain of no greater than 2 kg) and stable medication use for 6 months before enrollment" 时使用了过去完成时，其他地方都使用了一般过去时。

表 4-3　研究对象样例 1

Persons were eligible for inclusion if they were 65 years of age or older, were obese (body-mass index≥30), were sedentary (regular exercise <1 hour per week), and had had a stable body weight (loss or gain of no greater than 2 kg) and stable medication use for 6 months before enrollment. 15 persons who had severe cardiopulmonary disease (e.g., recent myocardial infarction or unstable angina), musculoskeletal or neuromuscular impairments that precluded exercise training, or cognitive impairments or who used drugs that affect bone metabolism were excluded.

在书写研究对象部分时，通常还需要详细描述研究对象的特征。

如果是以人为研究对象，应根据需要注明研究对象的人数（number）、性别（gender）、年龄（age/years)、体重（weight）、健康状况（health status）等详细情况。

如果是以实验动物为研究对象，需要注明动物的种类（species）、数量（number）、来源（origin）、性别（sex）、周龄（age/weeks）、体重（weight）、健康状况（health status）、饲养条件（feeding conditions）等基本信息。

如果是以细胞为研究对象，需要注明细胞的来源（origin）和培养条件（culture condition）等信息。

例如研究对象样例 2（表 4-4）中描述了实验动物的性别 female（雌性），种类 BALB/c mice（BALB/c 小鼠），周龄 6 to 8 weeks（6 到 8 周），实验动物的来源 from West China Experimental Animal Center（华西实验动物中心）。这一段中还描述了实验使用的细胞的种类 CT26 mouse colon carcinoma and 4T1 mouse breast carcinoma cells（CT26 小鼠结肠癌和 4T1 小鼠乳腺癌细胞），这两种细胞的来源 from the American Type Culture Collection（来自美国菌种收集中心），细胞的培养条件 cultured in RPMI 1640 supplemented with 10% heat-inactivated fetal serum and antibiotics（在添加了 10% 热灭活胎血清和抗生素的 RPMI 1640 培养基中进行培养）。

我们可以发现，这一段的两个句子都使用了一般过去时的被动语态。

表 4-4　研究对象样例 2

Female BALB/c mice, 6 to 8 weeks old, were purchased from the West China Experimental Animal Center. Both CT26 mouse colon carcinoma and 4T1 mouse breast carcinoma cells were obtained from the American Type Culture Collection and cultured in RPMI 1640 supplemented with 10% heat-inactivated fetal serum and antibiotics.

以人或以动物为研究对象的实验，都需要通过伦理审查、符合伦理学流程，从而获得权威认证机构授予的实验资质。并且需要在描述研究对象时（也可以在研究设计部分单独列出伦理审查部分）说明批准机构的名称、地点、时间、批准号等。另外，如果研究对象是人，还应该说明知情同意程序。

例如研究对象样例3（表4-5）中说明了该实验及后续实验均已通过伦理审查；说明了伦理审查机构名称：尼泊尔卫生研究委员会、莫纳什大学人类研究伦理委员会（the Nepal Health Research Council，the Monash University Human Research Ethics Committee），并注明了伦理批准号（reference number 1065/22854/1363）；还说明了所有参与者都提供了知情同意书（Written informed consent was obtained from all participants）。

表4-5　研究对象样例3

The trial was approved by the ethics review committee of the Nepal Health Research Council (NHRC; reference number 1065). The follow-up study was approved by the Monash University Human Research Ethics Committee (reference number 22854) and the NHRC (reference number 1363). Written informed consent was obtained from all participants in both the trial and the follow-up study.

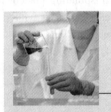

第四节
研究过程

在阐明研究对象之后，作者还需要详细说明具体的操作步骤，以便于读者重复操作，通常使用 Study procedure 或 Experimental procedure 等作为二级标题。研究过程是对方法部分第二语步"描述研究"的阐述，主要包含描述实验/研究程序，命名和描述用于测试或进行其他任务的工具，以及描述实验所测试的变量或进行实验的条件。

写作时需要明确研究过程中所采用的操作及测定方法（已发表但不为人

知的方法需提供参考资料及简要说明；描述新的或经过大幅度修改的方法时，给出使用它们的理由）；说明所使用的实验设备、试剂及材料等（注明型号、剂量、厂家等相关信息）。

例如研究过程样例（表4-6）中详细描述了研究所使用的方法和过程：所有受试者均接受常规标准治疗 → 患者随机分配到氟伏沙明组或相应的安慰剂组 → 研究人员为受试者提供欢迎视频 → 研究人员收集结果数据（All participants received usual standard care→Patients were randomly assigned to fluvoxamine…or corresponding placebo…→Researcher personnel provided participants with a welcome video…→Study personnel collected outcome data…）。研究过程中也说明了所使用药品（fluvoxamine）的种类（Luvox）、厂家（Abbott）和剂量（at a dose of 100 mg twice a day for 10 days）。

我们可以发现，这一段的句子既使用了主动语态，也用了被动语态，时态都用了一般过去时。

表 4-6　研究过程样例

All participants received usual standard care for COVID-19 provided by health-care professionals at public health facilities. Patients were randomly assigned to fluvoxamine (Luvox, Abbott) at a dose of 100 mg twice a day for 10 days or corresponding placebo starting directly after randomisation (Day 1). Research personnel provided participants with a welcome video, which gave information on the trial, study drug, adverse events, and follow-up procedures. Study personnel collected outcome data on Days 1, 2, 3, 4, 5, 7, 10, 14, and 28 in person or via telephone contact or social media applications using video-teleconferencing.

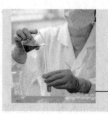

第五节
数据统计分析

作者在书写研究方法部分时，一般会描述研究所采用的统计学分析方法和过程，使读者能够通过原始数据来验证所报告的研究结果，从而建立研究的可信度。作为方法部分的第三语步"建立研究的可信度"，它通常包含准备数据、公布并描述统计工具和统计程序、说明所使用的统计规范、操作数据等步骤。

表 4-7 数据统计分析样例

All statistical analyses were performed using the Statistical Packages for the Social Sciences (IBM, SPSS Corp.; Armonk, NY, USA) Version 22 software. As appropriate to the nature of the parameters in the dataset, analyses were made using frequency tables, descriptive statistics, difference tests, and chi-squared tests. An independent samples T-test was used to calculate the differences between bi-categorical variables, and an F-test was used to calculate the differences between multi-categorical variables. In cases where the F-test indicated a significant difference, the least significant difference method was used post-hoc to determine which pair resulted in a significant difference. The level of statistical significance was considered to be 95 percent.

例如在数据统计分析样例（表4-7）的陈述中，作者告知了我们如下信息：

① 所采用的统计软件名称及版本：

SPSS Version22；

② 研究中所使用的统计方法：

frequency tables（频率表），descriptive statistics（描述性统计），difference tests（差异检验），以及 chi-squared tests（卡方检验）；

③ 采用这些统计方法的依据和标准：

An independent samples T-test was used to calculate the differences between bi-categorical variables（独立样本 T 检验是用来检验两分类变量间的差异），

an F-test was used to calculate the differences between multi-categorical variables（F 检验是用来检验多分类变量间的差异），

the least significant difference method was used post-hoc to determine which pair resulted in a significant difference（可以使用事后分析得出最小显著差异值，以判断哪两组之间的差异是显著的），

The level of statistical significance was considered to be 95 percent（统计的显著性水平被认定为95%）。

通过观察本段的时态和语态可以发现，每一句都使用了一般过去时的被动语态。

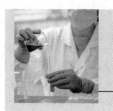

第六节
常用语法和句型

一、常用时态

医学研究型论文的方法部分中通常会使用一般过去时报告所采取的研究行为，表述所使用的研究对象、研究材料、研究方法、统计方法等发生在过去的操作，例如：

① Participants were recruited through advertisements and underwent comprehensive medical screening.

通过广告招募研究对象，并对其进行全面的医学筛查。

② The samples were frozen at –4℃ from the time of urine collection to the time of testing.

从尿液采集到检测，样品在 –4℃ 冷冻。

③ As appropriate to the nature of the parameters in the dataset, analyses were made using frequency tables, descriptive statistics, difference tests, and chi-squared tests.

根据数据中参数的性质，采用频率表、描述性统计、差异检验和卡方检验进行分析。

方法部分中通常会使用一般现在时解释或介绍标准研究工具、已经存在的数据或样本，描述行业规范或说明图表。例如：

① A typical chemical reactor includes a helical, tube-in-tube heat exchanger.

典型的化学反应器包括一个螺旋套筒式变温器。

② Clinicians providing usual care in public health facilities typically focus on the management of symptoms and provide antipyretics or recommend antibiotics only if they suspect bacterial pneumonia.

在公共卫生机构提供常规护理的临床医生通常侧重于症状管理，只有在怀疑细菌性肺炎时才提供退烧药或推荐抗生素。

③ The global study design is described in Fig. 1.

总体研究设计如图 1 所示。

有时方法部分也会使用过去完成时说明研究或实验之前已经发生的情况或已经完成的操作，表示这种情况或操作对研究或实验造成的影响。例如：

Persons were eligible for inclusion if they had had a stable body weight (loss or gain of no greater than 2 kg) and stable medication use for 6 months before enrollment.

体重稳定（减重或增重不超过 2 千克）并在之前稳定用药达 6 个月的参选者才能成为研究对象。

二、常用语态

自然科学研究型论文的方法部分中常用被动语态，并且往往会省略行为动作的发出者，从而强调研究方法、研究过程、研究对象、研究材料、研究数据的客观性。因此，在医学研究型论文的方法部分中使用被动语态的频率很高。例如：

① 使用被动语态表示研究对象的分组。

Participants were randomly assigned to a weight-management program or to a control group.

参与者被随机分配到体重管理组或对照组。

② 使用被动语态表示研究材料的选取。

Blood samples were collected on the day of colonoscopy, prior to the procedure.

在手术前的结肠镜检查当天采集了血液样本。

③ 使用被动语态表示研究数据的测定。

Levels of serum calcium, phosphorus, and magnesium were measured in patients.

对患者做了血清钙、磷及镁含量的测定。

从功能上来说，我们在方法部分使用被动语态是为了强调研究对象、研究材料、研究数据等客观对象。

有的情况下方法部分也会采用主动语态，比如在：① 需要将作者的方法和其他研究的方法区分开时；② 需要使段落中语态使用呈现多样性时，这两种情况下通常需要使用主动语态。

三、常用信号词

医学研究型论文方法部分涉及较多方面，因此，作者写作时可以参考使用以下信号词，以便于读者通过信号词了解方法部分结构和内容。

表 4-8　信号词

tests		carried out	adopted
samples		collected	applied
experiments		chosen	controlled
equipment		conducted	designed
drugs		administered	divided
models		generated	employed
instruments		obtained	extracted
materials	was/were	found in	filtered
participants		devised	included
control group		modified	installed
placebo group		performed	operated
patients		provided by	prepared
chemicals		purchased	recorded
apparatus		used	sampled
cells		investigated	scored
mice		measured	simulated
surgeries		selected	treated

我们也可以在方法部分的句子中加入表示研究目的的动词不定式结构"to+ 动词原型（见引言部分表 3-5）"，把研究目的和具体的研究方法步骤相结合，更易于读者理解。例如：

> To validate the results of the model, samples were collected from all age groups.
>
> 为了验证模型的结果，从所有年龄组收集了样本。

四、常用句型

① 表示前人使用的方法。

> Many researchers have used…to detect…
>
> Previously,…has been assessed by measuring…
>
> …is the most common method for examining…
>
> There are…types of …available for investigating…

② 表示本研究所采用的研究方法。

> Samples were analyzed for...as previously reported by...
>
> The study was approved by…
>
> Ethical approval was obtained from…
>
> ...was carried out by/using...as previously described
>
> ...was/were conducted/assessed/measured using the method...
>
> ...was prepared according to the procedure used by...
>
> ...was bred/fed in...
>
> ...was stained with...
>
> ...was grown in...medium.
>
> ...was treated/diagnosed by/with...

③ 表示采用该研究方法的原因。

> A major advantage of the method is that…
>
> …was used because it provides…
>
> The method is particularly beneficial in…
>
> The…approach was selected since/for…

…offers an effective way of…

④ 表示研究对象的选择及排除标准。

Criteria for selecting the subjects were as follows:

…who aged between…and…were included in...

Primary inclusion criteria for the participants were...

Exclusion criteria included...

...were excluded from the study if/ on the basis of...

...were considered ineligible for...

⑤ 表示研究对象的来源和分组。

The participants in this study were recruited from…

A random sample of patients with...was recruited from...

...were randomly selected among...

The cohort was divided/assigned into...groups according to/depending on...

The participants were divided/stratified/grouped into...groups based on...

...were randomized into...

...were randomly allocated to...

⑥ 表示材料来源。

...was/were obtained/purchased from...

...was/were donated/provided by...

⑦ 表示数据统计分析。

All analyses were carried out using SPSS, version...

The data were collected/ gathered from…

The data were normalized with…

…tests were carried out to determine whether...

A p value<0.05 was considered significant.

The level of statistical significance was considered to be 95 percent.

第五章

结果部分

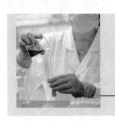

本章将探讨如何书写医学研究型论文的结果部分。论文中常用 Results 作为这一部分的标题，有时也可能会使用 Analysis 或者 Data Analysis。结果部分是论文正文的主体部分，这一部分通过文字、表格、图片等多种形式呈现研究数据，汇报研究结果，解答与回应引言部分所提出的研究问题及研究目的，并且给结论部分提供客观依据。论文的结果部分通常是最客观的一个部分，它向读者呈现未经修饰的研究数据，并且传达作者对结果的理解。

结果部分的主要写作内容包括：汇报研究数据（reporting data）和强调研究的主要发现（highlighting major findings）。特别需要注意的是，要避免罗列研究得到的所有数据，而要按照一定的逻辑顺序陈述有代表性的数据及主要的研究发现。常见的排列原则有：①按照引言部分所提出的研究问题及研究目的的顺序排列；②按照结果的重要性排列；③按照从概括到具体的顺序排列；④按照时间顺序排列。

除了根据以上排列原则有逻辑、有层次地描述研究结果，作者还可以像书写方法部分一样，添加一些二级标题，合理设置段落布局。比如临床医学研究型论文结果部分中常用的二级标题有：Operating parameters（手术参数），Efficacy（疗效），Primary outcome（主要结果），Secondary outcome（次要结果），Subgroup analyses（亚组分析），Complications（并发症），以及 Adverse events（不良事件）等。

在一篇医学研究型论文的结果部分中，几乎都会利用图表这种非常直观的形式呈现研究数据，但是用来描述结果的语言文字和图表一样不可缺少，甚至具有更重要的作用。因为图表中的数字或百分比并不能阐述其背后的含义，需要作者通过文字描述数据所代表的含义、比较数据间的差异、揭示数据之间的关联等，帮助读者通过阅读文字理解图表中的关键信号。例如句子

"As shown in Table 1, the side effect occurred in only 1% of patients"，作者通过 only 一词表达了 1% 的副作用是较低的，而这是无法通过图表表达的。

结果部分的结构和语步相较于其他部分来说更简单直接，不管是介绍什么方面的研究结果，通常都会包含三个语步（表 5-1）。第一语步中作者将读者的注意力引导到后面的文字或附带的插图或表格中。第二语步中作者以多种形式对研究得到的结果进行陈述。第三语步中作者对结果进行简单评价或与其他结果进行比较。

表 5-1　结果部分语步

语步 1：导入后续的文本或视觉元素（M1: import later text or visual elements）	
概括地呈现结果，提及并定位图表（可选）(present findings generally, and locate tables or figures)	例：The results of the correlational analysis are shown in Table 2. 相关性分析结果如表 2 所示。
语步 2：以不同形式呈现结果（M2: present results in different modes）	
以语言呈现（必选）(present in language)	例：The mean score for the group was 7.8. 这组的均值是 7.8。
以图表呈现（可选）present in figures or tables	略
语步 3：评述结果（M3: comment on results）	
评价或阐释结果（可选）evaluate or interpreting a result	例：As shown in Table 1 that the mortality rate in the Group 3 is the lowest. 如表 1 所示，组 3 的死亡率最低。
将结果和某物比较（可选）compare a result with something	例：From the data, a significant difference can be found between the two conditions. 从数据中可以发现两种病情之间存在显著差异。

表 5-2　结果部分样例

Mortality data are depicted in the form of Kaplan-Meier survival analysis (Figure 2). Multiple deaths occurred in the etanercept group after 30 days, in contradistinction to the lack of mortality in the placebo group after 30 days, thus accounting for the significant mortality difference observed at 6-month analysis. This observation is expanded in Table 5, which displays causes of deaths that occurred prior to 30 days and after 30 days in the two groups. The major causes of death in both groups included renal failure and hepatic encephalopathy.

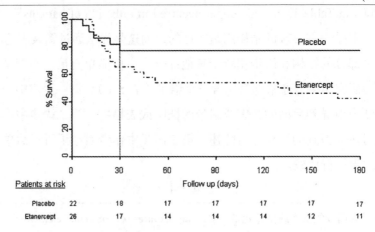

Figure 2. Kaplan Meier Survival Analysis
30-day mortality (vertical hashed line) was not significantly different between placebo (solid line) and etanercept (hashed line) groups. 6-month mortality rate was significantly higher in the etanercept arm compared to the placebo arm (p<0.05).

Table 5

Causes of death

	Placebo (n=5)		Etanercept (n=15)	
	Death within one month (n=5)	Death one through six months (n=0)	Death within one month (n=9)	Death one through six months (n=6)
Renal Failure	3	0	8	5
Sepsis	0	0	3	0
Hepatic encephalopathy	4	0	4	2
GI bleeding	2	0	2	1
Cardiopulmonary†	1	0	1	0

† Includes congestive heart failure and respiratory failure

‡ Note that some patients have multiple listed causes of death.

我们以表 5-2 中论文结果部分的一段为例，进一步了解结果部分的结构和语步。段落的第一句对应结果部分的第一语步"导入后续的文本或视觉元素"。在陈述由数据得到的研究发现之前，作者首先使用了一个引导句"Mortality data are depicted in the form of Kaplan-Meier survival analysis (Figure 2)"，引导读者结合表格进行该段落的阅读。

然后，作者开始撰写第二语步"以不同形式呈现结果"：以文中 Figure 2、Table 5（见表 5-2 末尾），以及文字的形式描述研究结果。第二句中前半句呈现了图 2 显示的结果"30 天后，依那西普组出现了多例死亡，安慰剂组没有出现死亡"后半句为第三语步"评述结果"，评述了前半句的研究结果"解释了 6 个月分析时观察到的显著死亡率差异"。

第三句"表 5 扩展了这一观察结果，显示了两组在 30 天之前和 30 天之后发生的死亡原因"，这一句其实也属于第一语步，引导读者观察表5中的数据结果。而最后一句中"两组的主要死亡原因包括肾衰竭和肝性脑病"属于第三语步，是基于表格中数据结果所作出的判断。

结合文中图表可以看出，作者并没有在段落中一一描述图表中的数据，而是将不同研究组间的数据进行比较之后，陈述作者通过数据所得到的研究发现。因此，作者在写作中要着重报告和研究主题及研究目的相关的数据结果，并通过语言文字阐述从图表中提炼出的重要研究发现。请比较两个句子：① The mean stone burden was significantly higher in patients who had multiple locations ($p<0.001$). ② The stone-free rates of patients who had distal stones and patients who had stones in multiple locations were different. 第一句基于结果部分的表格总结出了远端结石患者的无结石率明显高于多部位结石患者的无结石率；而第二句只是陈述了两组间的无结石率存在差异，但没有说明差异的程度是否显著、是否有意义，所以后者并没有完全揭示数据所能体现的重要信息。

在这个段落中，作者用一般现在时陈述第一语步，引导读者关注图表中的内容；用一般过去时描述第二和第三语步，回顾和总结研究结果和发现。

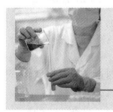

**第二节
常用语法和句型**

一、常用时态

结果部分多使用一般过去时和一般现在时，具体可以分为以下几种情况：

在段落中描述图表中提及的内容（例①②）或在图注和表注中进行陈述

说明时（例③），常用一般现在时。例如：

① Data of mortality are depicted in Kaplan-Meier survival analysis (Figure 3).

死亡率数据以 Kaplan-Meier 生存分析表示（图 3）。

② Patient screening and recruitment at each of the seven study sites are shown in Table 1.

七个研究地点的患者筛查和招募情况见表 1。

③ Note that some patients have multiple listed causes of death.

注意有些病人有多个所列出的死因。

描述医学上已被证明的常识时，通常使用一般现在时。例如下面两个例句中的前半句：

① Even with "per protocol" analysis, that is, only analyzing patients who received any injections, etanercept continued to be significantly associated with mortality.

即使采用"按方案"分析，即只分析接受任何注射的患者，依那西普也与死亡率显著相关。

② Because IL-6 and IL-8 are key cytokines downstream of TNF-α, baseline serum levels of IL-6 and IL-8 were assayed and are shown in Table 2.

由于 IL-6 和 IL-8 是肿瘤坏死因子 -α 的关键下游细胞因子，因此测定了 IL-6 和 IL-8 的基线血清水平，如表 2 所示。

结果部分内容大多是对于研究结果的回顾性陈述，因此在报告具体的研究数据或结果时，或在回顾所做的研究或研究发现时，常用一般过去时。例如：

① The stone-free rate was significantly higher in patients who had distal stones and lower in patients who had multiple locations ($p<0.001$).

远端结石患者的结石清除率显著高于多端结石患者 ($p<0.001$)。

② During the recruitment period, 174 patients were evaluated for enrollment.

招募研究对象期间，有 174 例患者接受评估后被招募。

说明之前的研究与本研究间的关系，或对本研究所造成的影响时，通常使用完成时态。例如：

Comparison of study patients with their age- and gender-matched healthy controls showed that study patients had significantly higher levels of IL-6 (79.7 ± 50.1 pg/mL vs 24.0 ± 8.4 pg/mL, respectively, p < 0.001) and IL-8 (52.6 ± 27.0 pg/mL vs 15.5 ± 26.9 pg/mL, respectively, p < 0.001) as has been previously reported.

正如先前的研究所报道的，与年龄和性别相匹配的健康对照组比较，研究组患者 IL-6 水平（分别为 79.7±50.1 pg/mL 和 24.0±8.4 pg/mL，p <0.001）和 IL-8 水平（分别为 52.6±27.0 pg/mL 和 15.5±26.9 pg/mL，p <0.001）显著升高。

二、常用信号词

结果部分写作过程中可能会用到一些信号词，见表 5-3。

表 5-3　结果部分常用信号词

名词	动词		形容词 / 副词	
figure	demonstrate	occur	brief(ly)	sufficient(ly)
table	show	produce	consistent(ly)	surprising(ly)
image	illustrate	reduce	important(ly)	expected(ly)
data	list	decline	Inadequate(ly)	unexpected(ly)
result	provide	drop	large(ly)	simple(ply)
analysis	reveal	change	low	noticeable(ably)
statistics	report	accelerate	main(ly)	satisfactory
tendency	indicate	affect	most(ly)	severe(ly)
majority	compare	improve	obvious(ly)	significant(ly)
frequency	find	present	only	similar(ly)
mortality	observe	correlate	remarkable(ably)	strong(ly)
incidence	suggest	predict	constant(ly)	same
morbidity	compare	confirm	different	very
death rate	rise	appear	higher	inconsistent
survival rate	increase	account for	highest	in line with
case	decrease	explain	lower	evident(ly)
value	imply	associate	insignificant(ly)	probably

(continued)

名词	动词	形容词 / 副词	
model		slightly	reasonable
		possible	logical

三、常用句型

结果部分没有固定的写作结构和书写顺序，因此会使用很多种句型，但经常使用到的句型有以下几种：

① 对应研究结果再次提及研究目的或研究方法。

The purpose of the experiment was to...

In order to investigate…was used.

As mentioned previously, the aim of the test was to…

In this step, we sought to…

② 概述结果。

In general, …

In this section, we evaluated/ compared/ reported…

The results are divided into…parts as follow:

③ 用来描述图表。

Table1/Figure 1 shows/demonstrates/presents (that)…

As shown in Table1/Figure 1, …

… is/ are shown/displayed/presented in Table 1/Figure 1.

As can be seen from/in Figure 1/ Table 1, …

From the table/ figure above/ below we can see that…

④ 用来具体描述结果（相似性）。

…is/are similar to…

…is/are consistent with…

…is/are in line with…

⑤ 用来具体描述结果（相关性）。

…was/were (positively/inversely/negatively) correlated/associated/connected with…

There was a relationship/correlation/association between A and B.

…was found to be correlated/associated with…

⑥ 用来描述显著差异。

There was significant difference between…and…

The difference between…and…was significant.

…was significantly different from…

⑦ 用来描述不显著差异。

There was no significant difference between…and…

No significant/Insignificant difference was found between…and…

⑧ 用来描述趋势变化。

…showed a tendency to increase.

…reminded steady/constant…

…increase/elevate/rise/decrease/reduce/ decline/drop by/to…

…range/vary from…to…/between…and…

⑨ 用来评价或阐释结果。

…may be due to…

…might be attributed to…

It could be inferred that…

This indicates that…

…may explain the correlation between…and…

⑩ 用来报告问卷或访谈结果。

The overall response to the survey was good.

There were 78 responses to the question.

The response rate was 68%.

71% of respondents reported/ said/ suggested that…

Some interviewees commented/ felt/ emphasized that…

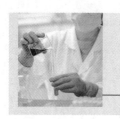

第三节
图表的有效利用

　　在书写医学研究型论文结果部分时，作者往往通过表格、插图等多种形式报告研究发现。表格和插图作为医学研究型论文的一个重要组成部分，可以直观地呈现支持研究结果的原始数据资料，客观地展示作者的研究成果，便于读者阅读、分析、获取信息。而文字能够阐述图表中数据所代表的意义，图表和文字相辅相成。因此，有效利用表格和插图中的信息是作者书写结果部分的关键。

　　首先，要了解什么时候需要在结果部分中使用表格和插图。表格用于容纳文本中过多或过于复杂的数据，以使文章更具可读性。当在结果部分中遇到复杂的数据（如实验数据、疾病的鉴别诊断、药物的不同作用等）时，我们可以将数据从段落中转移到表格里，使原本复杂的内容变得一目了然，便于分析比较，以增加文章的可读性。而插图可以直观生动地呈现研究结果，通常用于呈现结果数据的趋势、形式或者它们之间存在的关系，从而达到文字叙述难以达到的效果。

　　医学研究型论文中常见的表格类型有统计表、调查表、对照表等，其中以统计表最为常见。统计表一般采用三线表（图 5-1），即由 top line（顶线）、bottom line（底线）和 heading line（栏目线）构成的表格。

Top Line

Heading Line

Table 2. Hazard Ratios for Melanoma-Related Death, According to Multivariable Prognostic Factors.*				
Prognostic Factor	Dissection		Observation	
	Hazard Ratio (95% CI)	P Value	Hazard Ratio (95% CI)	P Value
Sex: male vs. female	1.13 (0.80–1.59)	0.50	1.41 (0.98–2.05)	0.07
Age, per 1-yr increase	1.00 (0.99–1.01)	0.93	1.01 (0.99–1.02)	0.15
Breslow thickness				
<1.50 mm†	1.00		1.00	
1.50–3.50 mm	1.64 (0.96–2.79)	0.07	2.46 (1.34–4.53)	0.004
>3.50 mm	3.82 (2.19–6.66)	<0.001	4.32 (2.31–8.09)	<0.001
Ulceration: present vs. absent	1.97 (1.40–2.77)	<0.001	2.17 (1.55–3.05)	<0.001
Site of melanoma				
Arm or leg†	1.00		1.00	
Head or neck	0.81 (0.44–1.48)	0.49	1.60 (0.96–2.66)	0.07
Trunk	1.26 (0.89–1.77)	0.19	1.05 (0.74–1.49)	0.80
No. of positive sentinel nodes				
1†	1.00		1.00	
2	1.08 (0.71–1.62)	0.73	1.27 (0.87–1.84)	0.21
≥3	1.17 (0.61–2.24)	0.64	2.01 (0.82–4.95)	0.13
Nonsentinel nodes: positive vs. negative	1.78 (1.19–2.67)	0.005	NA	

Bottom Line * Patients with positive findings on RT-PCR were excluded from this analysis. NA denotes not applicable.
† This group served as the reference group.

图 5-1　三线表样例分析 1

如图 5-2 所示，统计表一般是由 table No.（表序）、title（表题）、headings（栏目）、body（表体）、footnotes（表注）五个基本部分构成的。栏目按照方向又可以分为 vertical headings（纵向栏目）和 horizontal headings（横向栏目）。

Table No.

Horizontal Headings

Table 2. Hazard Ratios for Melanoma-Related Death, According to Multivariable Prognostic Factors.*				
Prognostic Factor	Dissection		Observation	
	Hazard Ratio (95% CI)	P Value	Hazard Ratio (95% CI)	P Value
Sex: male vs. female	1.13 (0.80–1.59)	0.50	1.41 (0.98–2.05)	0.07
Age, per 1-yr increase	1.00 (0.99–1.01)	0.93	1.01 (0.99–1.02)	0.15
Breslow thickness				
<1.50 mm†	1.00		1.00	
1.50–3.50 mm	1.64 (0.96–2.79)	0.07	2.46 (1.34–4.53)	0.004
>3.50 mm	3.82 (2.19–6.66)	<0.001	4.32 (2.31–8.09)	<0.001
Ulceration: present vs. absent	1.97 (1.40–2.77)	<0.001	2.17 (1.55–3.05)	<0.001
Site of melanoma				
Arm or leg†	1.00		1.00	
Head or neck	0.81 (0.44–1.48)	0.49	1.60 (0.96–2.66)	0.07
Trunk	1.26 (0.89–1.77)	0.19	1.05 (0.74–1.49)	0.80
No. of positive sentinel nodes				
1†	1.00		1.00	
2	1.08 (0.71–1.62)	0.73	1.27 (0.87–1.84)	0.21
≥3	1.17 (0.61–2.24)	0.64	2.01 (0.82–4.95)	0.13
Nonsentinel nodes: positive vs. negative	1.78 (1.19–2.67)	0.005	NA	

* Patients with positive findings on RT-PCR were excluded from this analysis. NA denotes not applicable.
† This group served as the reference group.

Title

Vertical Headings

Body

Footnotes

图 5-2　三线表样例分析 2

《生物医学期刊投稿的统一要求》中对论文中的表格有以下要求：

① Number tables consecutively in the order of their first citation in the text.

按照表格在正文中首次出现的先后顺序为表格标注阿拉伯数字序号。

② Supply a brief title for each table.

为每个表格提供一个简明扼要的标题。

③ Do not use internal horizontal or vertical lines.

表内一般不出现横线和竖线。

④ Give each column a short or an abbreviated heading.

给每栏一个简短的或缩写形式的标题。

⑤ The horizontal heading is generally used to indicate the objects and contents described in the table.

横向栏目一般用来表示表格所描述的研究对象和主要内容。

⑥ The vertical heading is generally used to illustrate the statistical indicators of each column.

纵向栏目一般用来说明各纵栏的统计指标。

⑦ Place explanatory matter in footnotes.

说明解释性的文字要置于表注中。

⑧ Explain all nonstandard abbreviations in footnotes, and use symbols (*, †, ‡, §, ||, ¶, **, ††, ‡‡) in sequence.

在脚注中解释表格中用规定符号标注的所有非标准缩写，并按顺序标注这些规定使用的符号（*、†、‡、§、||、¶、**、††、‡‡）。

医学研究型论文中常见的插图种类有示意图、统计图和照片图。示意图用来描述事物的性质或流程，统计图用来描述数据之间的关系，照片图则能够真实、直观地传递信息。医学论文中常用的示意图有结构图（structural diagrams）和流程图（flow charts）；常用的统计图有线图（line chart）、条图（bar chart）、饼图（pie chart）和直方图（histogram）等。

图 5-3 是统计图中的线图，主要由 figure No.（图序）、title（图题）、headings（标目）、lines（图线）、legends（图例）、footnotes（图注）等组成。和表格部分一样，我们也应该按照插图在正文中首次出现的先后顺序为其标注阿拉伯数字序号；也需要在图注部分对插图中出现的符号及缩写等给出说明性的解释。

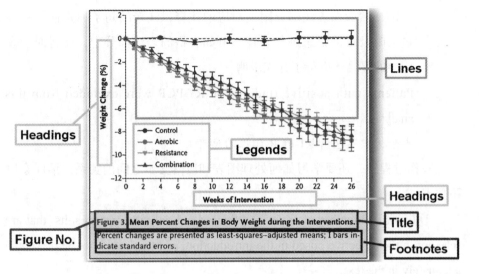

图 5-3 三线表样例 3

　　图表中的标题应力求简明扼要，标题的结构一般为名词性短语，尽量使用具有概括性的名词作为标题的重点词，通常要省去标题前的冠词。例如：

Characteristics of the Patients at Baseline

基线患者的特征

Prespecified Clinical Outcomes

预设的临床结果

Recruitment, Randomization, and Analysis Populations

招募、随机化和分析人群

除了图表标题，还要注意图表脚注部分的句子中所使用的时态。

① 在注明图表内某项内容时，通常要使用一般现在时。例如在图 5-1 中，作者使用一般现在时，对表格中出现的非标准缩略语 NA 进行了注释：NA denotes not applicable（NA 代表不适用）。

② 当需要在图表内提及研究中所使用的研究方法时，通常要使用一般过去时。例如图 5-1 和图 5-2 的表注部分中，结合符号标识出了参照组："This group served as the reference group." 因为作者对研究对象进行了分组，所以对照论文写作及发表时间来说，已经是过去时间，所以这里要使用一般过去时。

③ 另外，在对图表的标题进行说明、解释时，一般在标题后标注星号

上标，然后在表注部分附上对应的注释，注释的句子通常使用一般过去时及被动语态进行表述。例如表格的表注部分中，作者对应表题中的星号＊进行了补充说明。

Patients with positive findings on RT-PCR were excluded from this analysis.

本分析中不包括 RT-PCR 阳性的患者。

写作过程中，还要学习如何处理图表和段落文本之间的关系，请注意以下要点：

① Limit the number of tables and figures and only illustrate results that are relevant to the objective posed in the introduction, and that could not be presented adequately in the text.

如果遇到可以很容易地用文本总结的数据，就不需要使用表格或图表。尽量限制图表的数量，只有那些和引言部分提出的研究目的相关的，以及那些用文字无法恰当表达的研究结果，需要借助图表来呈现。

② Complement the tables and figures with text, but don't duplicate the same data.

用文本补充表格和插图，但要避免在文本中重复汇报图表中已经呈现的数据。

③ Number tables and figures separately and be sure all the tables and figures are referred to in the text.

表格和插图不能放在一起标序号，要分别标序，并确保在文本中提到论文中出现的所有图表。

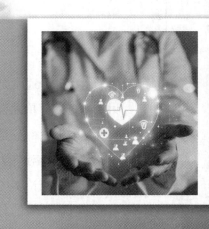

第六章
讨论部分

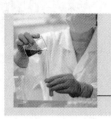

第一节
结构和语步

　　讨论部分通常是医学研究型论文正文的最后一个部分，有的期刊要求在讨论部分后面单独设置结论部分。期刊中常用 Discussion 作为这个部分的英文标题。讨论部分是作者总结、评估和解释本研究结果，从中得出推论和结论，并传达其对科学和社会贡献的部分。

　　作为一篇论文的重难点部分，讨论部分相比论文的其他部分而言，往往最能够反映作者的分析能力和科研写作水平。论文结果部分的主要内容是展示研究数据，而讨论部分的主要任务是对这些结果数据进行解释。当研究结果和作者预期结果有很大差异时，在讨论部分解释这样的研究结果对于作者来说就更具挑战性了。

　　讨论部分的写作要紧扣引言部分所提出的研究目的，作者要以结果部分为依据，对研究发现进行合理的解释，总结研究结论并探讨研究的价值。不同期刊、不同医学研究领域对于讨论部分的结构可能会有特定的要求，但通常情况下讨论部分的结构都可以分为以下三大语步及其中的若干写作步骤（表6-1）。

　　讨论部分的第一语步中作者通常会明确研究人员实施了实验，达到了研究目的或者回答了研究问题（比如：We conducted…to investigate the effect of…），并简要概括主要的研究发现（比如：This study found that…）。

　　讨论部分的第二语步内容更加丰富，是讨论部分非常重要而不可或缺的一个语步。这个语步中作者将本研究的发现与前人的研究发现进行对比（比如：Our findings are similar to those of… 或 The present study differs from previous studies in…），并对本研究的发现进行解析（比如：A possible explanation for this finding may be…）。只有将本研究和前人研究进行比较，才能凸显本研究的贡献。如果本研究和前人研究结果一致，说明本研究进一步有效证明了前人的研究发现；如果本研究和前人研究结果不一致，说明本研究有新的发现和突破。除此之外，作者还需要对本研究的发现给出合理的解释，尤其解释与先前研究不同的发现或与研究假设相悖的发现。

讨论部分的第三语步对研究进行总结，讨论研究发现在该医学研究领域中所产生的作用和意义（This study offers some insight into...），说明本研究因为研究方法等因素而产生的局限性（比如：Some limitations of the current study are...），并对未来的研究给出一些建议（比如：What needs to be investigated further is...）。作者一般会在陈述研究贡献后，讨论研究的局限性并给出相关建议，这可以让读者及审稿人了解本研究的不足，增强研究结果的可信度，也给作者或同领域的研究人员指出未来研究的方向。

表 6-1　讨论部分语步

语步 1（M1）：重述研究发现（restate the research outcome generally）

　步骤 1（S1）：重述研究目标（restate the objective of the study）

　步骤 2（S2）：总结主要研究发现（summarize the major findings）

语步 2（M2）：详细回顾和解释研究发现（review and explain the findings in detail）

　步骤 1（S1）：将本研究的发现与以前其他相关研究的发现进行比较
（compare the findings with previous studies）

　步骤 2（S2）：解释研究发现，尤其是意料之外的发现
（interpret the findings, especially the unexpected findings）

语步 3（M3）：总结研究（summarize the study）

　步骤 1（S1）：讨论本研究的意义（discuss the implications of the study）

　步骤 2（S2）：说明本研究的局限性（state the limitations of the study）

　步骤 3（S3）：建议进一步研究的方向（recommend the direction of further research）

现在以一篇医学研究型论文的讨论部分为例（表 6-2），具体说明讨论部分的写作。这篇论文介绍了儿童特应性皮炎与睡眠质量的关系，其研究目的是"To determine whether children with active atopic dermatitis have impaired sleep duration and quality at multiple time points throughout childhood and whether disease severity affects sleep outcomes."（确定患有活动性特应性皮炎的儿童在整个儿童期的多个时间点上的睡眠时长和质量是否受损，以及疾病的严重程度是否影响睡眠的效果。）

表 6-2 讨论部分样例

Among the 13,988 children from the ALSPAC cohort followed up from birth through adolescence, we found similar sleep duration between Children with active atopic dermatitis and those without. In contrast, children with active atopic dermatitis experienced worse sleep quality throughout childhood. This association was the largest among children with more severe disease and among children with asthma or allergic rhinitis, but it remained statistically significant even for those with inactive and mild disease.

These findings are consistent with those of small cross-sectional studies of clinic populations that used objective measures of sleep, including actigraphy and polysomnography. In those studies, despite increases in sleep fragmentation and reductions in sleep efficiency, overall sleep duration was similar between children with and without atopic dermatitis.[6-10]

In contrast, time spent awake after sleep onset is consistently greater among children with atopic dermatitis, ranging from approximately 45 to 100 minutes.[6-9] In addition to increased nighttime awakenings and difficulty falling asleep, we found that children with active atopic dermatitis were more likely to report nightmares and early morning awakenings, which has not been previously studied.[10]

Children with inactive disease still reported increased odds of impaired sleep quality, at a level similar to those with active but mild disease. Moreover, scratching episodes only accounted for 15% of the arousals and awakenings, suggesting that scratching alone does not explain the sleep fragmentation experienced by these patients. Fishbein and colleagues[5] have proposed that this phenomenon may be associated with a heightened sensitivity to sensory stimulation at night secondary to skin damage, which may represent an underlying mechanism of hyperarousability despite good disease control.[6,29] Other factors that may be implicated in atopic dermatitis–associated sleep disturbances include cytokine and melatonin dysregulation and disrupted circadian rhythms of the skin.[30]

This study has several limitations that warrant discussion. As in all large-scale longitudinal studies, the study was missing data and attrition occurred over time. For this reason, we repeated the analyses after conducting multiple imputation and found that the results were similar, which helped address concerns of potential selection bias. Another important limitation was the possibility for misclassification bias because both exposure and outcomes were parent- or self-reported.

Notwithstanding these limitations, this study has several implications for future research and clinical care. Currently, only a few atopic dermatitis clinical outcome measures address sleep and may not adequately capture the extent of sleep quality disturbances.[44,45] Our findings support the development of standardized and validated clinical outcome measures of sleep disturbance that explicitly address several aspects of sleep quality.[45,46] This refinement would enable future trials to assess the effectiveness of atopic dermatitis interventions in reducing poor sleep.

讨论的第一段中，作者重申了研究的四项主要发现：① "we found similar sleep duration between children with active atopic dermatitis and those without."（我们发现活动性特应性皮炎儿童和非活动性特应性皮炎儿童的睡眠时长相似。）② "children with active atopic dermatitis experienced worse sleep quality throughout childhood."（研究发现患有活动性特应性皮炎的儿童在整个儿童期的睡眠质量较差。）③ "This association was the largest among children with more severe disease and among children with asthma or allergic rhinitis,"（这种联系在患有更严重疾病的儿童和患有哮喘或过敏性鼻炎的儿童中最为显著。）④ "but it remained statistically significant even for those with inactive and mild disease."（但即使对那些病情轻微的患儿来说，这种联系也具有统计学意义。）

作者在这一部分中重申了本研究的主要研究结果，但并未重复结果部分的语句，这点是值得关注和学习的。因为读者在讨论部分之前刚刚阅读过结果部分，所以作者需要换一种方式阐释、总结研究发现，而不是单纯地重复。我们看到作者重述了每一项重要发现，并通过过渡语 In contrast 和 but 将这四项重要发现连接起来。另外，文中使用了一般过去时简要总结研究结果。

概述了研究结果之后，作者在第 2~3 段中将本研究的研究结果和前人的相关研究结果进行了比较。第 2 段说明本研究和前人的一些研究存在结果上的一致性。"These findings are consistent with those of small cross-sectional studies of clinic populations."（这些研究发现与对临床人群进行的小范围横断研究的研究结果一致。）结果的一致性存在于 "…overall sleep duration was similar between children with and without atopic dermatitis."（本研究和前人的这些研究都发现患有和未患有特应性皮炎的儿童的整体睡眠时间是相似的。）

第 3 段中，作者首先陈述本研究与其他研究相一致的研究发现 "…time spent awake after sleep onset is consistently greater among children with atopic dermatitis"（特应性皮炎患儿入睡时间更长，也就是入睡更困难。）然后重点陈述前人研究中所未发现的 "…children with active atopic dermatitis were more likely to report nightmares and early morning awakenings"，（本研究发现患有活动性特应性皮炎的儿童更容易出现噩梦和清晨醒来的情况。）

这几段和前人研究的比较中，作者使用 are consistent with 和 is consistently greater among 来表示不同研究间在研究结果上存在的一致性，并且使用一般现在时来描述这种具有普遍意义的事实；使用现在完成时 has not been previously studied 陈述前人尚未研究发现的问题；而对于研究结果的陈述 "we found that…were more likely to…"，作者依然使用一般过去时。

在第四段中，作者就一些主要研究发现进行了解释。作者首先陈述研究结果，"Children with inactive disease still reported increased odds of impaired sleep quality, at a level similar to those with active but mild disease. Moreover, scratching episodes only accounted for 15% of the arousals and awakenings…" 患有非活动性特应性皮炎的儿童睡眠质量受影响的概率增加，其水平与那些患有轻度活动性特应性皮炎的儿童相似，抓挠时长只占微觉醒和觉醒时长的 15%。之后作者解释了研究结果所代表的含义 "suggesting that scratching alone does not explain the sleep fragmentation experienced by these patients"，（这表明抓挠并不能完全解释这些患儿所经历的睡眠片段化。）我们看到，作者使用了 suggesting 一词来引导从句，阐释结果数据背后的深层含义。并且，作者还通过引用文献解释了为什么会出现这种结果，指出有以下几种因素可能会引起患儿睡眠的片段化，这些因素分别是 "a heightened sensitivity to sensory stimulation at night secondary to skin damage"（继发于皮肤损伤的在夜间对于感官刺激的高度敏感性），"cytokine and melatonin dysregulation"（细胞因子和褪黑激素的失调），以及 "disrupted circadian rhythms of the skin"（皮肤生理节律的紊乱）。

作者使用了 this phenomenon may be associated with, other factors may be implicated in 来表示对于可能会引起患儿睡眠障碍的影响因素的推测，may be 这种模糊语（hedges）的使用加强了学术语篇的严谨性。

第五段中作者讨论了本研究的局限性。作者以一个主旨句引导段落 "This study has several limitations that warrant discussion."（这项研究有几个值得讨论的局限性）。其中的第一个局限性在于 "As in all large-scale longitudinal studies, the study was missing data and attrition occurred over time."（与所有大规模的纵向研究一样，这项研究也会随着时间的推移而出现数据的流失和损耗）。本研究的另一个局限性在于 "the possibility for misclassification bias because both exposure and outcomes were parent- or self-reported."（可能会出现错误分类偏倚的情况，因为结果都是由父母或研究对

象自己报告的）。对应所提出的局限性，作者还提出了他们在研究过程中是如何克服局限因素的。

作者使用一般现在时陈述了这项研究存在着局限性的事实，而在具体回顾研究过程中所存在的局限性是什么时，使用了一般过去时。

第六段中作者阐述了本研究的意义。在陈述研究意义之前，作者用了一个过渡句将研究的局限性和研究意义进行衔接"Notwithstanding these limitations, this study has several implications for future research and clinical care."（尽管存在这些局限性，本研究对未来的研究和临床治疗还是有一些启示的）。之后再具体阐述两方面的研究意义：① "Our findings support the development of standardized and validated clinical outcome measures of sleep disturbance that explicitly address several aspects of sleep quality."（我们的发现支持了对睡眠障碍进行的标准化和有效的临床结果测量的发展，在几个方面明确地解决了睡眠质量问题）；② "This refinement would enable future trials to assess the effectiveness of atopic dermatitis interventions in reducing poor sleep."（这一进步将使未来的实验能够评估对特应性皮炎进行干预治疗在减少不良睡眠中的有效性）。

作者在陈述研究意义时使用了一般现在时，并且使用情态动词 may 和 would 这类模糊语表达作者谨慎的态度。

这篇论文讨论部分的语步包括：对主要研究发现的概述、与相关研究结果进行的比较、对主要研究结果的解释、对研究局限性的陈述以及对研究意义的讨论。在书写讨论部分时，我们要根据研究内容设计讨论部分的写作结构，也可以添加项目标题，使结构更加清晰。

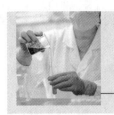

一、常用时态

讨论部分中可能会需要使用到多种时态，需要通过大量阅读文献，发现其中的使用规律。

① 在讨论部分，一般使用过去时来总结研究结果。

Our randomized, controlled trial involving obese adults 65 years of age or older indicated that weight loss plus a combination of aerobic and resistance exercise improved physical function and reduced frailty more than weight loss plus aerobic exercise or weight loss plus resistance exercise.

我们的随机对照实验对象为 65 岁及以上的肥胖成年人，结果表明，与减重加有氧运动或减重加阻力运动相比，减重加有氧运动和阻力运动结合能改善身体功能，减少虚弱程度。

② 当作者解释结果或描述发现的意义时，一般使用现在时。

Our results provide important implications for the better control of liver cancer.

我们的研究结果为更好地控制肝癌提供了重要的启示。

③ 在讨论部分的句子中，通常会同时使用过去时和现在时。

63% of the children demonstrated an elevated level of at least one risk factor, indicating that children with obesity are at an increased risk of cardiovascular diseases.

63% 的儿童表现出至少一种风险因素水平升高，这表明肥胖儿童患心血管疾病的风险增加。

前半句指的是结果，因此，这部分使用了过去时。后半句中使用现在时，用来说明前半句中所陈述结果代表的含义。

④ 作者在讨论部分中为进一步的研究提出建议或提供未来的研究方向时，可能需要使用将来时。

The methods reported here will open up avenues for further research in the field.

这里报道的方法将为该领域的进一步研究开辟道路。

二、常用信号词

作者书写讨论部分时可以参考表 6-3 中的信号词。

表 6-3　讨论部分常用信号词

表示比较	表示贡献与意义		建议未来研究方向
	形容词	动词	
consistent with	advantage	enhance	future work
consistency	convincing	facilitate	further study
contrast	effective	help	should be explored
in line with	efficient	improve	recommend
different from	feasible	be able to	remain to be
in agreement with	important	provide	advise
similar to	novel	support	promising
like	valuable	solve	be needed
in accordance with	significant		urgent
accord with	useful		possible
better	valid		

三、常用句型

作者在书写讨论部分时，可以参考使用以下句型。

① 用于重述研究目标、总结研究结果。

The purpose of this study was to gain a better understanding of …

The results of the present study support the hypothesis that …

There are three key findings of the present research. First … Second … Third …

In conclusion/general/summary, from the investigation of…, we found that…

② 用于解释研究结果。

One interpretation of these findings is that…

This finding may be explained by…

A possible explanation for this might be that...

This result/inconsistency may be due to/explained by/attributed to...

These results are likely to be related to...

These conflicting experimental results could be associated with...

...be responsible for...

...may lead to/result in/account for...

...may be caused by...

③ 用于将本研究的结果与以前其他相关研究的结果进行比较。

The result is consistent with the previous studies… (citation).

...is similar to the findings of previous studies.

These results match those observed in earlier studies.

These results are in accord with previous studies indicating that...

These results are in agreement with those obtained by...

In accordance with previous studies, our study has demonstrated...

However, this result has not previously been described.

The result is contrary to the hypothesis/previous studies which have suggested that...

The findings of the current study do not support the hypothesis/previous research.

The result differs from the findings of...

Our results are different from...

Contrary to the previous studies/our hypothesis...

④ 用于探讨本研究的意义。

Despite these limitations, these results suggest several theoretical and practical implications.

These results/findings have important implications for...

The study offers insights into···

These findings may/will/might/should help us to...

The findings of this study provide a new understanding of...

The experiments/results/findings/investigations supply a basis for...

There is of great significance in.../to...

⑤ 用于说明本研究的局限性。

There are several potential limitations concerning the results of this study.

A first limitation concerns... A second potential limitation is that...

One limitation of this study is that...

Although..., it is important to recognize several potential limitations.

Certain limitations of this study could be addressed in future research...

Our study has some limitations, for example, we only concentrate/focus on...

⑥ 用于给未来研究提出建议或方向。

Our study raises some questions for future study.

In terms of future research, it would be useful to extend the current findings by examining...

There is a need for future research that explores...

Further work/research/studies/investigations is/are needed/required to identify/establish/confirm/assess/determine/evaluate/explore...

More research on this topic needs to be done to...

Further analysis/experiments will be necessary to...

Further research on... may shed light on...

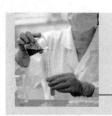

对模糊限制语的定义可追溯到元话语（metadiscourse）的概念。这一概念由 Harris 提出，是能够促进语篇的衔接及连贯的语言素材，能够协助作者表达观点、引导读者，能够帮助读者对语篇中呈现的信息进行组织、分类、理解及评价，从而促进作者和读者以语篇为媒介进行交流。

Hyland（2005）构建了包含引导式元话语和互动式元话语两个维度的元话语模式（表6-4），其中引导式元话语强调语篇组织功能，帮助作者理解语篇，互动式元话语将读者带入其中，强调人际交流功能。

表 6-4　元话语人际关系模式（Hyland, 2005）

引导式元话语（interactive metadiscourse）		
种类	功能	举例
过渡语 (interactive)	表达句子之间的关系	in addition; but
框架标记 (frame markers)	表示语篇界限和结构	finally; to conclude
内指标记语 (endophoric markers)	指向语篇的其他部分	in section 2
言据标记 (evidentials)	表明信息或观点来源	according to X
语码释义 (code glosses)	进一步解释命题意义	namely; such as
互动式元话语（interactional metadiscourse）		
种类	功能	举例
模糊限制语 (hedges)	保留观点和开启对话	might; perhaps
强化语 (boosters)	强调确定性或关闭对话	definitely; in fact
态度标记语 (attitude markers)	表达作者对命题的态度	agree; fortunately
介入标记语 (engagement markers)	与读者建立联系的显性手段	you can see that
自我提及 (self-mentions)	文中明确的作者自我指称	I; we; our

元话语的应用研究多以学术语篇为载体。学术论文写作中不仅需要传达科学的客观性，同时也需要表明作者严谨的学术态度及与同行进行交流的意愿。

在医学领域，作者希望可以尽可能全面、准确和客观地呈现信息，但由于很多医学研究存在样本量小、检测技术不完善或在实验过程中存在不确定因素等，学术写作过程中作者需要在事实和评估之间寻找平衡。因此，作者经常说"X may cause Y"而不是"X causes Y"来准确并留有余地地说明该主题的实际知识状态。模糊限制语可以帮助作者区分实际的和潜在的、已知的和推论的事物。

医学研究型论文的讨论部分中，作者要面向读者解释研究发现、比较研究发现、分析研究意义和局限性，以及建议未来研究方向。模糊限制语可以帮助作者表明接纳不同学术声音和观点的意愿，同时也用来对自己的学术观点持一定保留态度。作者通过使用模糊语，对所表达的学术观点持谨慎的态度，一定程度上弱化陈述语气，以避免因激进或过度自信的语言而影响自己或他人的学术声誉。讨论部分在表明主观看法、提出建议时，常用情态动词作为模糊限制语，例如：This information could also serve as a valuable reference for other cancer preventive vaccines.

这一句中使用了情态动词 could 表达作者的主观看法，作者认为这个信息也可以为其他癌症预防疫苗提供有价值的参考。

作者通常可以借助以下模糊限制语谨慎表达学术观点和主张（表6-5）：

表6-5 常用模糊限制语

类别	模糊限制语	举例
动词	about, appear, assume, estimate, feel, seem	Although the results seem to support previous findings…
情态助动词	can, could, may, might, should, would	The experiments may not represent…
形容词	estimated, likely, unlikely, probable, possible, presumable, doubtful, supposed, typical, uncertain	It is likely that the experimental group…
副词	approximately, around, generally, largely, mainly, mostly, perhaps, possibly, probably, presumably, relatively, roughly, typically	The number of patients will probably increase.
短语	from ×'s perspective, in general, in most cases, in ×'s opinion, in ×'s view, tend to	From our perspective, the disagreement could be attributed to…

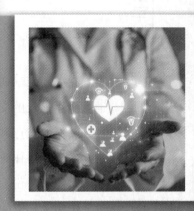

第七章
文内引用

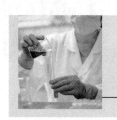

在书写医学研究型论文，尤其是论文的文献综述部分时，作者通常需要通过引用前人的文献来为本研究提供支撑。除了已经被广泛接受的事实或真理，其他的观点和事实都需要通过引用前人文献作为支撑。因此，引用文献是学术研究写作无法避免的环节，它可以展示作者的学术诚信、表明作者的学术素养和身份、表达对前人研究贡献的认可和尊重、为读者提供在该领域进一步阅读研究的参考来源。

医学研究型论文中通常在引言、方法和结果部分引用文献，通常可以分为以下几种情况（Bahadoran et al., 2020）。

表 7-1　论文不同部分引文的作用

引言部分	提炼有关研究问题的背景资料
	显示与研究问题相关的当前知识
	显示前人如何研究该问题
	呈现与研究问题相关的概念和变量
方法部分	描述前人的研究方法或标准规范
	描述复杂或鲜为人知的统计分析
	定义研究中使用的诊断标准
	合理化样本量估计
	解释研究设计或方法的合理性
结果部分	（没有引用）
讨论部分	将本研究结果与其他研究作比较
	反映当前对研究问题的各种看法
	支持可能的解释和含义
	给研究发现提供背景支撑

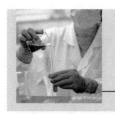

为了避免抄袭（plagiarism），作者需要将前人文献中的句子合理融入自己的研究论文中，因此需要掌握在文内引用文献（in-text citation）的技能。根据写作需要，一般有三种文内引用方法：直接引用（quoting）、改写（paraphrasing）和概述（summarizing）。

一、直接引用

直接引用指引用论文中的原句，并加上引号。有几种方法可以将引用的原句融入论文。通常情况下，比起直接引用整个长句，将原句中较为简短的一部分引入作者书写的句子中效果会更好，例如：During the 1970s, the U.S. began what has now become known as the "war on drugs", a reaction to the counterculture and drug-fueled climate of the 1960s. 当然也可以直接引用完整的长句，例如：Kidder (2003) noted that "providing sick people with medicine, but no food, is like washing one's hands and drying them off in the dirt." 然而，在写作中不应过度使用直接引文，在可能的情况下，尽量使用改写和总结的方法引用文献，用作者自己的语言解释想要引用的原文。

二、改写

改写指作者使用自己的语言转述所引用文献中的原句，使其与原文不同，但保留原有的含义。

例1：

（原文1）Symptoms of the flu include fever and nasal congestion.

流感的症状包括发烧和鼻塞。

（改写1）Stuffiness and elevated temperature are signs of the flu.

鼻塞和体温升高是流感的症状。

例2：

（原文2）Although white rice accounts for 35%~80% of the caloric intake for 3.3 billion Asians, it has several problems, such as lack of adequate nutrition, which makes Asian's body size relatively small; and also a lack of taste, which leads to high consumption of sodium in many of the foods eaten with rice.

虽然白米占33亿亚洲人热量摄入的35%~80%，但它存在几个问题，如缺乏足够的营养，这使得亚洲人的体型相对较小；而且味道也不好，就需要很多配菜，导致钠的摄入量很高。

（改写2）Lack of nutrition and taste in white rice leads to small body size and over-consumption of sodium of Asians respectively.

白米缺乏营养和口感，分别导致亚洲人体型偏小和钠摄入过量。

很显然，改写句子比直接引用文献中的句子困难，但也有一些技巧。比如可以通过使用同义词（如将 show 改为 demonstrate）、改变动词形式（如把主动语态改为被动语态）、改变词性（如把动词改为名词）或使用不同的句子结构进行转述。

三、概述

与直接引用和改写相比，当作者不需要提供所引用文献的细节内容，只需要大致描述文献的主要内容或观点时，可以使用概述（summarizing）的方式引用文献。概述是用作者自己的语言概括引用文献的要点，省略可能分散读者注意力的细节或例子，并简化复杂的语法、词汇和观点。例如：

（原文）Traditional medicine, which uses a wide variety of inexpensive, easily accessible, and familiar natural ingredients and techniques, is preferable for many people. Traditional medicines are normally created from local plants, animals, and minerals. Techniques often include socially bonding physical contact between patient and healer like rubbing or massaging, and spiritual experiences which may involve trances, music, and scents. In Africa, for instance, an estimated 80% of people rely on traditional medicine for almost all their health care. Similarly, in many other parts of the world, particularly in Asia and Latin America where modern facilities are available, this approach to medicine is still highly valued because it is effective, inexpensive, and culturally significant.

（概述）Traditional medicine is more popular in many places of the world because of its effectiveness, low cost and cultural value.

虽然改写和概述都是作者对所引用文献的理解和阐释，但两者还是有以下区别的：

表 7-2　改写和概述的区别

改写	概述
准确阐述引用的内容	简要概括引用的内容
通过重新措辞阐述原意	通过简要介绍概括大意
保留细节	省去细节
和原文相比长度相似或略短	明显比原文短

在使用概述的方法总结文献时，作者通常可以遵循以下步骤：

① 阅读文献中需要引用的文献，画出关键词及短语；

② 写下你画线的单词及短语；

③ 在不看原文的情况下，写一到两句话概括大意；

④ 对于每一个论点，都用一到两个句子进行总结；

⑤ 把所写的句子组合成一个段落；

⑥ 校对这个段落，检查有无错误或重复；

⑦ 将这个段落引入本文献。

总之，作者在写作中引用文献时，应首先仔细阅读文献，发现被引文献与本研究之间的特定关联，确定可以直接引用的、需要改写的以及需要概述的内容，以支撑自己的写作。

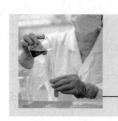

第三节
引文标注分类

　　无论作者采用以上哪种方式引用文献，都必须在引文处注明原文出处。医学研究型论文的引文标注方式主要有以下三种。

一、以信息为中心

　　以信息为中心（information-focused）指在引文句末加括号标注引用文献的作者姓名和论文发表年份（例 1）；或者在引文句末标注对应的参考文献编号，并通过字体设置为"上标"的形式（例 2）。这种标注方式优先显示引文信息而不是作者信息，更强调引文的内容。

　　例 1：

　　Tuberculosis is a disease that is more commonly found in individuals living in poverty, and it is also a cause of extreme socioeconomic stress. (Reid et al., 2019)

　　结核病是一种常见于生活贫困人群的疾病，也是造成极端社会经济压力的一个原因。(Reid et al., 2019)

　　例 2：

　　Tuberculosis is a disease that is more commonly found in individuals living in poverty, and it is also a cause of extreme socioeconomic stress.[17]

　　在引用文献时，作者可能需要引用多篇在某一方面具有相似点的文献，比如这些文献可能采用了相似的研究方法、研究角度，得出了相似的研究结果等，这种情况下作者就可以采用以信息为中心的标注方法，强调所引文献在内容和主张上的相似性。例如，以下句子阐述了该论文的参考文献 1 和 2 的共同点"evaluated outcomes at a young age"，文献 4 和 5 的共同点"a short observation period"，和文献 6-9 的共同点 "a small sample size"。

例 3：

Studies to predict the development of obesity on the basis of childhood BMI have suggested a positive correlation, but most have evaluated outcomes at a young age[1,2] or have had a relatively late baseline evaluation,[3] a short observation period,[4,5] or a small sample size.[6-9]

二、以作者为中心

以作者为中心（author-focused）是指把作者姓名放在引文句子的主语位置，并在作者姓名后加括号注明出版年份。这种标注方式凸显了引文作者在该领域的作用及学术地位。例如：

Sudfeld and colleagues (2020) found that although vitamin D3 was well tolerated, there was no effect of vitamin D3 supplementation on the risk of mortality.

Sudfeld 等 (2020) 发现，尽管维生素 D3 耐受性良好，但补充维生素 D3 对死亡风险没有影响。

表 7-3 罗列了以信息为中心和以作者为中心标注引文的区别。在医学研究型论文中常用以信息为中心的引文标注方式，因为自然科学研究更强调所引用文献的客观研究发现，较少强调所引文献中作者的观点和思想。

表 7-3 以信息为中心和以作者为中心标注引文的区别

以信息为中心（Information-focused）	以作者为中心（Author-focused）
突出被引内容，削弱被引者学术话语权	突出被引作者，强化被引者学术话语权
概括多方来源相同或相似的内容或主张	呈现单一来源的内容或主张
帮助本文作者控制所引内容或主张	过多使用可能会削弱本文作者的地位
节约更多文本空间	占用更多文本空间
建议常使用	需谨慎使用

三、以作者为中心的弱化形式

以作者为中心的弱化形式（weak author-focused）是指在引文句子中使

用"研究者"（Researchers）等较为宽泛的身份词来代替作者的名字，并在引文句末加上对应的参考文献编号（例 1），或加括号标注引用文献的作者姓名和论文发表年份（例 2）。该形式介于以作者为中心（author-focused）的方式和以信息为中心（information-focused）的方式之间，弱化了引文作者的作用。例如：

例 1：

Researchers suggest that for every week delay in diagnosis or treatment, mortality is increased by more than 1%.[4]

研究人员表示，诊断或治疗等每延迟 1 周，死亡率就提高 1%。[4]

例 2：

Researchers indicate that increased levels of carbon dioxide in the atmosphere are reducing levels of nutrients (such as zinc, iron, calcium, and potassium) in wheat, barley, potatoes, and rice. (Myers et al., 2014)

研究人员指出，大气中二氧化碳含量的增加正在减少小麦、大麦、土豆和大米中营养物质（如锌、铁、钙和钾）的含量。(Myers et al., 2014)

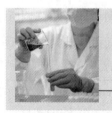

第四节
常用表达方式

一、常用报告动词

在医学研究型论文中，作者通常会在引用文献时使用报告动词（reporting verbs）描述所引作者的行为。这些报告动词可以分为以下三种类型（表 7-4）。

表 7-4　按照行为分类报告动词

研究行为 （research）	analyze, conduct, demonstrate, examine, find, investigate, test, observe, show, study…
认知行为 （cognition）	assume, advocate, acknowledge, believe, consider, expect, imply, hypothesize, think, hold, notice, support, speculate…
话语行为 （discourse）	argue, announce, assert, claim, comment, conclude, criticize, discuss, indicate, note, report, remark, suggest, state, object…

另外，作者在使用这些报告动词阐述引用文献时，也表明了其不同的立场（stance），比如作者通过使用 acknowledge, establish, remind (us), establish 等报告动词表明对所引内容或观点的接受和认同；使用 describe, present, demonstrate, show 等表达对所引内容或观点的中立态度；使用 claim, assert 等表示对所引内容或观点持保留态度。

二、常用句型

根据文内引用的不同方式和标注方法，作者可以参考使用以下常用句型：

① 直接引用句型。

As Swales states/points out/argues/concludes: "…" (Swales, 2024)

According to sb. "…" (Swales, 2024)

② 引用单一文献。

Swales' study (2024) found that…

Swales et al. (2024) reported/showed/found/demonstrated that…

A recent study by Swales (2024) described…

In a study conducted by Swales (2024), it was shown that…

X, Y and Z appear to be closely linked (Swales, 2024)

③ 引用多个文献。

Many recent studies (Smith, 2023; Swales, 2024) have shown that…

A number of researchers have investigated the effects of…(Smith, 2023; Swales, 2024)

To date, several studies have examined the association between... (Smith, 2023; Swales, 2024)

Previous studies of…have established…(Smith, 2023; Swales, 2024)

Previous studies have failed to find any significant differences in... (Smith, 2023; Swales, 2024)

The causes of…have been widely investigated…(Smith, 2023; Swales, 2024)

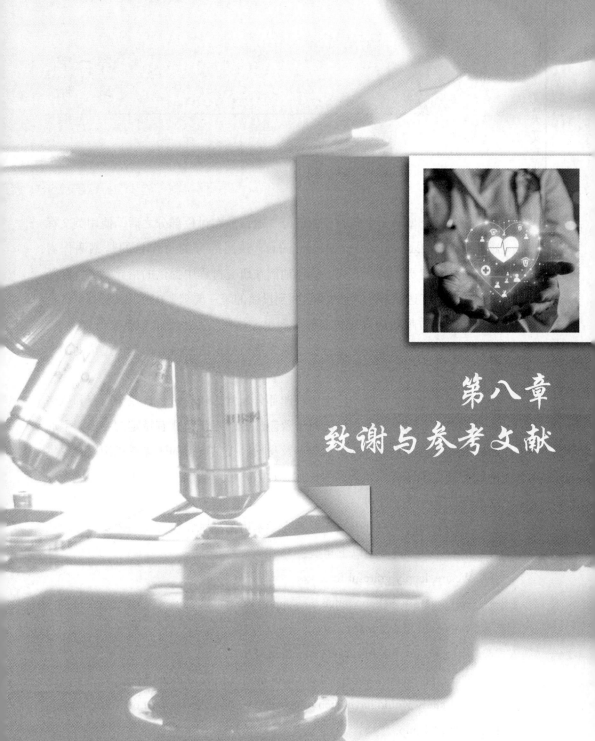

第八章
致谢与参考文献

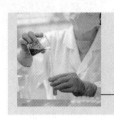

　　医学研究型论文中若有致谢部分，通常放在讨论部分之后，使用英文标题 Acknowledgement/Acknowledgements。致谢部分的写作目的是感谢作者之外对研究有贡献的所有人，感谢他们在研究过程中提供的指导、支持和帮助，向他们表达敬意。《生物医学期刊投稿的统一要求》中指出：所有不符合作者标准的贡献者都应在致谢部分列出，这些贡献者可能包括在研究设计、材料设备、数据收集、数据分析、论文撰写或论文修改方面提供过帮助的个人或团体。

　　相比学位论文，期刊论文的致谢部分通常比较简短，且致谢内容和风格更为严肃。不同医学期刊可能对于致谢部分的写作格式有特定的要求，但通常内容都会包括贡献者的个人全名及身份、提供支持的团体或机构以及提供的资金或物质支持。如果罗列贡献者姓名，可以按照贡献大小罗列，或者按照姓名首字母顺序排列。

　　研究论文的致谢部分写作要遵守学术道德准则，语言简明扼要、专业严谨、重点突出，常使用以下句型：

　　We are deeply grateful for…

　　We gratefully acknowledge the support of…

　　We would like to thank…for…

　　The research for this article was funded by…

　　The experiment was carried out with the… project funded by…

　　This study would have been impossible without the support of …Foundation/scholarship/Group.

　　下面我们通过两个样例进一步了解致谢部分写作。表 8-1 致谢部分样例 1 中，第一段的第一句中作者感谢一些机构对研究的资助。第二句中作者感谢研究所提供的分子和其他服务。第二段中作者对参加临床试验的患者及其家属、参与试验操作规划的公司、提供制图协助的公司以及为手稿的早期版本提供医学写作支持的 Advait Joshi 博士表示感谢。

表 8-1 致谢部分样例 1

Acknowledgments

Supported by Amgen, a Cancer Center Core Grant (P30 CA 008748 [to Memorial Sloan Kettering Cancer Center]), an M.D. Anderson Cancer Center Support Grant (P30 CA016672), a Clinical Translational Science Award (1UL1 TR003167), and a grant (RP150535) from the Cancer Prevention Research Institute of Texas Precision Oncology Decision Support Core. The Sheikh Khalifa Bin Zayed Al Nahyan Institute for Personalized Cancer Therapy provided molecular and other services.

We thank the patients and their families for participating in the trial; Maya Shehayeb, Pharm.D., Timothy Harrison, Pharm.D., and Jennifer Martucci, B.F.A. (all employed by Amgen), for operational planning assistance; Robert Dawson, B.A., for graphics assistance; and Advait Joshi, Ph.D., of Cactus Life Sciences (part of Cactus Communications) for medical writing support with an earlier version of the manuscript.

表 8-2 致谢部分样例 2 第一句中作者感谢了参与本研究的患者及其家属和护理人员，以及所有研究人员和研究机构的工作人员。第二句感谢了 Kevin Norwood 等 Merck Sharp & Dohme 公司员工。第三句感谢了 Charlotte Majerczyk 博士提供的医学写作和编辑协助。最后一句向资助这些协助服务的公司致谢。

表 8-2 致谢部分样例 2

ACKNOWLEDGMENT

The authors thank the patients and their families and caregivers for participating in this study, along with all investigators and site personnel. The authors also acknowledge the contributions of Kevin Norwood, Lei Xu, Susan Zeigenfuss, Janine Mahoney, Nathan Sciortino, Shawn Crockem, Tammy Winser, Galina Kourteva, all employees of Merck Sharp & Dohme Corp., a subsidiary of Merck & Co., Inc. (Kenilworth, NJ). Medical writing and editorial assistance were provided by Charlotte Majerczyk, PhD, of C4 MedSolutions, LLC (Yardley, PA), a CHC Group company. This assistance was funded by Merck Sharp & Dohme Corp., a subsidiary of Merck & Co., Inc., Kenilworth, NJ.

从以上两个致谢样例中可以发现，致谢通常使用一般现在时（比如 We thank the patients and their families for…），但如果是陈述研究过程中所得到的资助，通常使用一般过去时（比如：This assistance was funded by…）。

第八章 致谢与参考文献

81

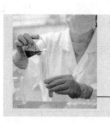

作者除了在文内引用文献以引导读者了解研究背景体系，还应该向读者提供所引用文献的详细信息，对所引文献的作者表示尊重，同时也可以帮助读者更有效地检索这些文献。

参考文献是医学研究型论文不可缺少的重要组成部分，标题通常为Reference。常见的参考文献类型包括期刊论文、学位论文、会议论文、著作、科学技术报告、网页文章等。

参考文献通常应按文中首次提及的顺序连续编号，也有的期刊按照第一作者姓名字母顺序排列。论文参考文献的格式通常因所投期刊而异，也因所参考文献的类型而异。医学期刊论文常用参考文献格式有如下3种，表8-3中详细列举了这3种参考文献格式。

APA：美国心理学会（American Psychological Association）的《美国心理协会刊物准则》，多应用于心理学领域、语言学、社会学等社会科学领域。

AMA：美国医学会（American Medical Association）出版的参考文献格式，广泛应用于医学和生物学领域，尤其是美国医学会出版的期刊中。

NLM：美国国家医学图书馆（National Library of Medicine）出版的参考文献格式，通常用于医学、生物学及相关领域，是国际医学期刊编辑委员会（ICMJE）推荐的格式。

表 8-3　常用参考文献格式

	APA
期刊论文	Author, A. A., Author, B. B., … (Year). Title of article. *Title of Periodical*, volume number (issue number), pages. DOI. 第一作者姓，第一作者名前缀，第二作者姓，第二作者名前缀……（发表年份）. 论文标题. *期刊名称*，卷号（期号），页码. 数字对象唯一标识符. 例: Shah, S. C., & Itzkowitz, S. H. (2022). Colorectal Cancer in Inflammatory Bowel Disease: Mechanisms and Management. Gastroenterology, 162(3), 715–730.e3. https://doi.org/10.1053/j.gastro.2021.10.035.
著作	Author, A. A. (Year of publication). *Title of work*. Edition Number. Publisher. 作者姓，作者名前缀（出版年份）. *著作标题*. 版次号. 出版商名称. 例: Brownson, R. C. (2011). Evidence-based Public Health. 2nd ed. Oxford University Press.
网页文章	Author, A. A. (Year, Month Date). Title of page. Site name. URL. 作者姓，作者名前缀 .（年，月，日）. 页面标题. 网站名. 网址 例: Schmidt, C. (2024, 2, 12).New Research Shows Little Risk of Infection from Prostate Biopsies. Harvard Health Blog. https://www.webmd.com/diet/foods-rich-in-potassium.
	AMA
期刊论文	Author, A. A., Author, B. B.,…Title in sentence case. *Abbreviated Journal Title in Title Case*. Year; volume number (issue number): Pages. DOI. 第一作者姓，第一作者名前缀，第二作者姓，第二作者名前缀，……（用句首大写方式表示的论文标题. *词首字母大写的期刊标题缩写*. 年；卷号 (期号): 页码范围. 数字对象唯一标识符. 例: Paredes F, Williams HC, San Martin A. Metabolic adaptation in hypoxia and cancer. Cancer Lett. 2021;502:133-142. doi:10.1016/j.canlet.2020.12.020.
著作	Author, A. A. *Title of work*. Edition Number. Place of Publication, Initials of Publication Place: Publisher;Year of publication. 作者姓，作者名前缀 . *著作标题*. 版次号 . 出版城市，出版城市单词首字母: 出版社名称；出版年份 . 例: Brownson, RC. Evidence-based Public Health. 2nd ed. New York, N.Y.: Oxford University Press; 2011.

网页文章	Author, A. A. Page title. Website Name. Published Month Day, Year. Accessed Month Day, Year. URL. 作者姓，作者名前缀 . 页面标题 . 网站名 . 发布月日，年 . 引用月日，年 . 网址 . 例： Pelc C. Prescription steroids affect brain structure, study finds. Published September 6, 2022. Accessed September 8, 2022. https://www.medicalnewstoday.com/articles/prescription-steroids-affect-brain-structure-study-finds.

NLM

期刊论文	Author, A. A., Author, B. B.,…Title in sentence case. *Abbreviated Journal Title in Title Case*. Year + Month Abbreviation + Day; volume number (issue number):Pages. DOI. 第一作者姓，第一作者名前缀，第二作者姓，第二作者名前缀，……(用句首大写方式表示的论文标题 . *词首字母大写的期刊标题缩写* . 年 + 月份缩写 + 日；卷号 (期号): 页码范围 . 数字对象唯一标识符 . 注：期刊名称缩写参考美国国家医学图书馆（NLM）网站 例： Lilly AC, Astsaturov I, Golemis EA. Intrapancreatic fat, pancreatitis, and pancreatic cancer. *Cell Mol Life Sci*. 2023 Jul 15; 80(8):206. doi: 10.1007/s00018-023-04855-z.
著作	Author, A. A. *Title of work*. Edition Number. Place of Publication: Publisher; Year of publication. Pagination. 作者姓，作者名前缀 . 著作标题 . 版次号 . 出版城市 : 出版社名称；出版年份 . 页数 . 例： Eyre HJ, Lange DP, Morris LB. *Informed Decisions: the Complete Book of Cancer Diagnosis, Treatment, and Recovery*. 2nd ed. Atlanta: American Cancer Society; 2002. 768 p.
网页文章	Author, A. A. Website Name [Internet]. Place: Publisher; Published Month Day, Year. [Date of Update/Revision/Citation]. Available from: URL. 作者姓，作者名前缀 . 网站名 [Internet]. 地点 : 出版商 . [更新 / 修订 / 引用日期]. 网址 . 例： Huckstep RL, Sherry E. World Ortho [Internet]. [place unknown: publisher unknown]; [updated 2007 Mar 23; cited 2007 Mar 23]. Available from: http://www.worldortho.com/.

对应文末参考文献，有的期刊要求作者在正文中以（作者姓氏＋发表年份）的方式引用参考文献，有的期刊要求作者在正文中以对应文末参考文献顺序的数字加上标的方式引用参考文献（例如[1]），具体要参考计划投稿的期刊。文内引用的详细方法可以参考"文内引用"章节中的描述。

除了参考文献的格式，作者在选择参考文献时还应遵循以下原则：

① 尽量引用原始参考文献，并对照原始文献核实参考文献信息是否有误或者是否已被撤稿。

② 避免过多地引用自己的文献。

③ 避免过多地引用同一期刊来源文献。

④ 避免使用摘要作为参考文献。

⑤ 避免引用个人交流信息，除非该交流提供了无法从公开来源获得的重要信息，在这种情况下，应征得交流人的书面许可，并应在正文的括号中注明交流人的姓名和交流日期。

⑥ 引用已被接受但尚未发表的论文时，应获得书面许可，并确认其已被接受发表，应注明"in press"（出版中）或"forthcoming"（即将出版）。

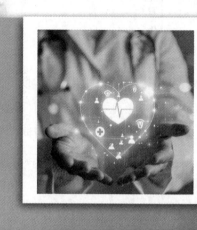

第九章
摘要和关键词

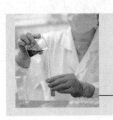

国际医学期刊中医学研究型论文的摘要部分一般位于论文的标题页之后、正文之前，是对研究内容的概括，向读者提供论文正文中的关键信息。读者通过主题词检索到感兴趣的文献之后，通常会首先阅读文献摘要，再决定是否阅读整篇文献。因此，写好英文摘要可以将医学研究成果介绍给全世界更多的读者，在国际医学领域进行交流。

虽然摘要通常排版在论文正文前，但作者应在书写完正文部分后，再进行摘要部分的写作。《生物医学期刊投稿的统一要求》中说明，摘要中应提供研究的背景，说明研究的目的，描述研究所采用的方法，陈述主要的研究发现及研究结论。

基于这一要求，医学研究英语论文的摘要一般会采用报道性摘要（informative abstract）来描述这些信息。按照格式，报道性摘要可以分为非结构式摘要（non-structured abstract）和结构式摘要（structured abstract）两种类型。

非结构式摘要采用的是传统的一段式摘要。表 9-1 中就是一篇非结构式摘要。其中 "The smoking habit of 48 patients with malignant hypertension was compared with that of 92 patients with non-malignant hypertension." 描述了研究所采用的方法：将 48 例恶性高血压患者与 92 例非恶性高血压患者的吸烟习惯进行对比研究。"Thirty-three of the patients with malignant and 34 of the patient with non-malignant hypertension were smokers when first diagnosed, the differences were considered significantly." 描述了研究发现：初诊时就已吸烟的恶性高血压患者有 33 例，非恶性患者 34 例，两者之间有显著性差异。"Results suggest that malignant hypertension is yet another disease related to cigarette smoking." 阐述了基于研究结果所得出的研究结论是：恶性高血压是

一种与吸烟有关的疾病。非结构式摘要使用完整句，读者需要仔细阅读来分辨段落中所包含的层次。

表 9-1　非结构式摘要样例

Abstract: The smoking habit of 48 patients with malignant hypertension was compared with that of 92 patients with non-malignant hypertension. Thirty-three of the patients with malignant and 34 of the patients with non-malignant hypertension were smokers when first diagnosed, the differences were considered significantly. Results suggest that malignant hypertension is yet another disease related to cigarette smoking.

相较于非结构式摘要，结构式摘要是更加结构化、规范化、标准化的报道性摘要。表 9-2 中的摘要就是结构式摘要，它以清晰的结构罗列出 objective（目的）、methods（方法）、results（结果）、conclusions（结论）这些子项目名称，就每个项目展开简要叙述。

表 9-2　结构式摘要样例

Abstract

Objective: To determine the impact of body mass index (BMI) in adulthood or childhood on the reproductive health of women.

Methods: Heights, weights (at 7, 11, 16, 23 and 33y) and reproductive data were available for 5799 females in the British cohort study in 1958. Body mass index (BMI) was calculated as weight/height. Age-specific cut-offs were used to define overweight and obesity. Reproductive problems reported at age 33 included: menstrual problems (also reported at 16y), hypertension in pregnancy and subfertility.

Results: Early menarchal age was associated with menstrual problems by 16y, but the relationship did not persist to 33y. After adjusting other interference factors, obesity at both 23y and 7y are associated with menstrual problems before 33y (OR=1.75 and 1.59 respectively). Obesity at 23y increased the risk of hypertension in pregnancy (OR=2.37). Consistent with these findings, obese women at 23y were less likely to conceive within 12 months of unprotected intercourse (RR=0.69).

Conclusions: Overweight and obesity in early adulthood seems to lead to menstrual problems, hypertension in pregnancy and subfertility. Other than menstrual problems, childhood body mass index had little impact on the reproductive health of women.

并不是所有的结构式摘要都由这四个部分构成，有的医学期刊的摘要中还会包含 background（背景）、design（研究设计）、setting（研究地点）、participants（研究对象）、main outcome measures（主要测定项目）等子项目。

例如，著名医学期刊 *The New England Journal of Medicine*（新英格兰医学杂志）的常用摘要结构是由 background（背景）、methods（方法）、results（结果）、conclusions（结论）四个项目构成的。*The Lancet*（柳叶刀）的常

用摘要结构包含 background（背景）、methods（方法）、findings（结果）、interpretation（解释）、funding（经费）这五个层次。而 BMJ（英国医学杂志）的常用摘要结构包含 objective（目的）、design（设计）、setting（研究地点）、participants（研究对象）、interventions（干预措施）、main outcome measures（主要测定项目）、conclusions（结论）七个项目层次。总的来说，结构式摘要便于编辑、审稿、检索及阅读，因此，很多国际医学期刊都要求作者采用这种形式来撰写摘要。

在撰写摘要的时候，还要遵循以下原则：

① consistency：要保证摘要的内容与论文正文内容的一致性。

② conciseness：要注意语句的简洁性，一篇摘要通常只有 200~300 个单词，或只占据一页，因此要避免出现冗余的信息，比如："This paper discusses two issues." 这句话就比较多余。

③ objectiveness：要保证摘要的客观性，避免使用具有主观色彩的表达，比如 very much, extremely, absolutely 这样具有主观色彩、对程度界定非常模糊的词，不应该出现在摘要中。

④ no tables or figures, no references: 摘要中通常不要添加图表，也无需标注引文。

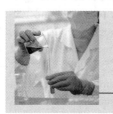

第二节
摘要的背景和目的部分写作

作者在摘要部分写作中通常需要回顾与研究相关的背景（background），以引出研究问题或目的。摘要的背景部分所陈述内容通常包括医学常识、论文主题、相关研究现状或者相关研究发现等。表 9-3 中例 1 使用一般现在时陈述了与研究相关的医学常识。例 2 使用现在完成时描述了与本研究相关的前人的研究发现，可以使用 …has/have been reported/shown/presented 句型进行表述。

表 9-3　结构式摘要背景部分样例

① Background: Surgical intervention is needed in some cases of spontaneous abortion to remove retained products of conception.

背景：在一些自然流产的病例中，需要进行手术来移除残留的妊娠产物。

② Background: Testosterone supplementation has been shown to increase muscle mass and strength in healthy older men. The safety and efficacy of testosterone treatment in older men who have limitations in mobility have not been studied.

背景：对于年龄较大且活动量有限的男性，补充睾酮可以增加肌肉量和增强肌力。

③ BACKGROUND & AIMS: The incidence of hepatocellular carcinoma (HCC) increases with age, but protective antibody response decreases with time after infants are immunized against hepatitis B virus (HBV). We investigated whether immunization of infants against HBV prevents their developing HCC as adults.

背景和目的：肝细胞癌的发生率随着年龄的增长而增加，而婴儿接种乙肝病毒疫苗后，保护性抗体反应随时间的推移而降低。我们调查研究了婴儿接种乙肝疫苗是否能预防他们成年后发生肝细胞癌。

有时候作者会在背景部分提出研究问题。比如表 9-3 ②，作者在第一句中描述了"补充睾酮可以增加年龄较大且活动量有限的男性的肌肉量以及增强其肌力"的研究发现，接着在第二句中提出了有待在本研究中解决的问题。可以使用 sth has/have not been studied，There are few studies on sth 或者 It is not known whether... 等句型描述研究问题。

作者也可以在背景部分提出研究目的。③的第一句中陈述了一个医学常识"肝细胞癌的发生率随着年龄的增长而增加，而婴儿接种乙肝病毒疫苗后，保护性抗体反应随时间的推移而降低"。然后提出了本研究的目的"我们调查研究了婴儿接种乙肝疫苗是否能预防他们成年后发生肝细胞癌"。

作者在摘要的目的部分提出论文要探讨、解决的问题或进行科学研究的理由。非结构式摘要和结构式摘要中目的部分的写作方法是不同的。在非结构式摘要中，我们需要用完整句表述研究的目的。表 9-4 的四句完整句中使用了 The purpose of this paper is to...，The aim of our study was to...，The study was designed to...，We aimed to... 等常用句型表达研究目的，并且使用了一般过去时。

表 9-4　非结构式摘要目的部分样例

① The purpose of this paper was to describe the clinical presentation of 30 such patients.

撰写本文的目的是介绍 30 例该类患者的临床表现。

② The aim of our study was to determine whether there is a significant difference in the results of both treatments.

进行本研究的目的是确定两种治疗方法的结果是否具有显著性差异。

③ The study was designed to investigate whether acute infections transiently increase the risk of venous thromboembolism.

设计本研究的目的是研究急性感染是否会暂时增加静脉血栓栓塞的风险。

④ We aimed to determine whether outcomes in patients with acute ischemic stroke could be improved by positioning the patient to be lying flat during treatment to increase cerebral perfusion.

我们想确定急性缺血性脑卒中患者在治疗过程中，通过使患者平躺以增加脑灌注，是否可以改善预后。

　　而在结构式摘要中，目的部分通常使用项目标题 Objective，Aims 或者 Purpose 加上动词不定式短语进行表达，这样更加简练。例如：

　　Objective: To determine the optimum interpregnancy interval after miscarriage in a first recorded pregnancy.

　　目的：探讨首次有记录的妊娠流产后再次妊娠的最佳时间间隔。

　　另外，除了项目标题 Objective 的首字母要大写，动词不定式标记 to 的首字母也要大写。医学研究型论文结构式摘要中常用于表示目的的动词不定式有：to observe（观察）、to compare（比较）、to determine（确定）、to develop（研发）、to evaluate（评价）、to investigate（调查）、to study（研究）等。

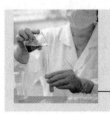

第三节
摘要的方法部分写作

　　在结构式摘要中，作者通常用 Methods 作为方法部分的项目标题，也有的结构式摘要会用 design、setting、participants、outcome measurements and statistical analysis 等项目标题，更为细致地陈述研究所使用的方法。

摘要方法部分概括地介绍了研究设计、研究对象、研究材料、实验方法、数据的测定方法以及数据的统计方法等信息。比如表 9-5 中描述了研究采用访谈的方法（We interviewed...）；描述研究对象选取和分组的方法：分别选取了 622 名新近被诊断为肝细胞癌的患者以及 660 名健康对照者（600 patients newly diagnosed with HCC...along with 660 healthy controls...）；描述所测定的研究数据：研究对象在肝细胞癌发生前或登记作为对照者前不同年龄阶段的体重、身高和体型（weights, heights, and body sizes at various ages before HCC development or enrollment as controls）；描述研究所采用的数据统计及计算方法：采用多变量逻辑回归分析和 Cox 回归分析，并计算出体重指数（Multivariable logistic and Cox regression analyses were performed...BMI was calculated）。

表 9-5　摘要方法部分样例

> **METHODS:** We interviewed 622 patients newly diagnosed with hepatocellular carcinoma (HCC) from January 2004 through December 2013, along with 660 healthy controls to determine weights, heights, and body sizes at various ages before HCC development or enrollment as controls. Multivariable logistic and Cox regression analyses were performed to determine the independent effects of early obesity on risk for HCC and patient outcomes, respectively. BMI was calculated, and patients with a BMI of 30 kg/m^2 or greater were considered obese.

摘要的方法部分通常使用一般过去时对已经发生的研究操作过程进行回顾和总结。并且方法部分常使用被动语态表示研究对象的分组（例如：Participants were randomly assigned to a weight-management program or to a control group. 参与者被随机分配到体重管理项目组或对照组）；表示研究材料的选取（例如：Blood samples were collected on the day of colonoscopy, prior to the procedure. 在结肠镜检查当天，即手术前采集血样）；表示研究数据的测定（例如：Levels of serum calcium, phosphorus, and magnesium were measured in patients. 对患者做了血清钙、磷及镁含量的测定），从而强调研究对象、研究材料、研究数据等客观对象。

在国际医学期刊中，在方法部分使用主动语态描述研究所采用的研究设计、实验方法的情况也很多。使用主动语态时，句子的主语常用第一人称复数形式 We 代表整个研究团队，例如 We conducted a trial...（我们进行了一项试验）；We stratified patients…（我们对患者进行了分组）；We collected data…
（我们收集了数据）。

摘要方法部分的常用词汇和句型可以参考第四章内容。

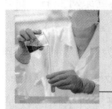

第四节
摘要的结果和结论部分写作

结构式摘要中通常使用 Results 作为结果部分的项目标题，也有的期刊
会使用 Findings。结果部分通过实验测出的重要数据、患者的治疗结果或统
计学处理结果等，描述本研究的主要研究结果。表 9-6 这段摘要的结果部分
中陈述了"成年早期肥胖是肝细胞癌的重要危险因素"的研究结果，并分别
统计出整体人群中、男性中和女性中的成年早期肥胖率。统计结果表明，成
年早期体重增加与肝细胞癌诊断年龄的减小有显著的相关性。研究还发现肥
胖与肝炎病毒感染之间的协同作用，及肥胖对肝细胞癌患者的总体生存率没
有影响。

表 9-6　摘要结果部分样例

RESULTS: Obesity in early adulthood (age, mid-20s to mid-40s) is a significant risk factor for Hepatocellular Carcinoma (HCC). The estimated odds ratios were 2.6 (95% confidence interval [CI], 1.4–4.4), 2.3 (95% CI, 1.2-4.4), and 3.6 (95% CI, 1.5–8.9) for the entire population, for men, and for women, respectively. Each unit increase in BMI at early adulthood was associated with a 3.89-month decrease in age at HCC diagnosis ($P < .001$). Moreover, there was a synergistic interaction between obesity and hepatitis virus infection. However, we found no effect of obesity on the overall survival of patients with HCC.

结果部分也是回顾性陈述，因此通常使用一般过去时。摘要结果部分
常用词汇和句型可参考正文写作部分结果章节。要注意的是，摘要中使用
"The results showed that/ The results demonstrated that/ 或 The results suggested
that…"等句型表达结果时，通常会省略前面的内容而直接陈述 that 后面所

要表达的结果，使结果更加简洁易懂。

结构式摘要中通常使用 Conclusions 作为结论部分的项目标题。结论部分一般要求作者基于研究目的、结合研究结果集中阐述研究的理论或应用价值，其主要内容包括总结研究结果、分析研究结果、评价研究意义及局限性、展望今后的研究方向。例如表 9-7 这一段摘要的结论部分中第一句总结了研究结果："以结肠镜检查为参考标准，对全血样本中自然杀伤细胞活性进行检测，发现结直肠癌患者的敏感性为 87.0%，阴性预测值为 99.4%"。第二句对不同研究对象的研究结果进行了比较分析："与自然杀伤细胞活性高的受试者相比，自然杀伤细胞活性低的受试者患结直肠癌的风险要高 10 倍"。而最后一句评价了研究的临床意义："该试验可用于临床实践中，以评估患者罹患结直肠癌的风险。"

表 9-7　摘要结论部分样例

Conclusions: Using colonoscopy as the reference standard, a test for natural killer (NK) cell activity in whole blood samples identified patients with colorectal cancer (CRC) with 87.0% sensitivity and a negative predictive value of 99.4%. Subjects with low NK cell activity had a 10-fold higher risk of CRC compared with subjects with high NK cell activity. This test might be used in clinical practice to assess patients for risk of CRC.

摘要结论部分常用词汇、句型及语法时态等可参考论文正文中的讨论部分。

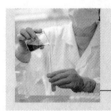

第五节
关键词

并不是所有国际医学期刊的研究论文都罗列关键词。如果期刊要求罗列关键词，通常要求书写在英文摘要之后，使用"Key Words"作为项目标题。在选用关键词时要遵守以下原则。

首先，关键词代表与论文主题内容相关的主题词（subject headings），也是文献检索的索引词（index words）。因此，在选择关键词时，常常会从论文标题和摘要中选择涉及研究主题、研究目的、研究对象以及研究手段的核心词汇。例如表 9-8 中论文标题是"妊娠早期糖尿病肥胖患者的身体活动、妊娠体重增加：一项随机对照试验"，它的关键词"妊娠期糖尿病，身体活动，肥胖，妊娠"均和论文主题相关。

表 9-8　英文关键词样例

Physical activity, gestational weight gain in obese patients with early gestationaldiabetes: A randomized–controlled trial
Keywords: Gestational diabetes mellitus, Physical activity, Obesity, Pregnancy

其次，选择英文关键词时一般要选用名词或名词性词组，而不选择动词、形容词等。例如 Treatment（治疗）、Obesity（肥胖）等名词，或 Clinical trial（临床试验）、Metabolic syndrome（代谢综合征）等名词性词组。为了便于文献检索，英文关键词要尽量使用专业词汇，尽量不要使用含义极其宽泛的词，比如 Diagnosis, Treatment 等，尽可能采用美国国立医学图书馆编辑的医学主题词表（Medical Subject Headings，MeSH）中所列的名词或名词词组。

最后，在书写英文关键词时，还应该注意以下书写格式：①选用 2~5 个关键词，最多 10 个；②每个关键词的首字母大写；③相邻关键词之间以逗号或空格相隔；④作者应按所投医学期刊具体要求书写英文关键词。

第十章
投稿信函

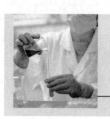

投稿（submission）是论文发表（publication）前极其重要的一个阶段。它并不是一个随意而轻松的过程，相反，按照期刊要求提交初稿，并在顺利进入修改环节后按要求认真修改，是一个相当艰巨的过程（详见图10-1）。

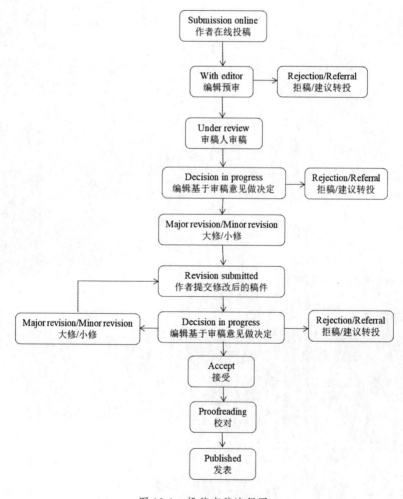

图 10-1　投稿审稿流程图

完成初稿之后，首先要选择目标期刊。选择过程中，作者应考虑：①目标期刊在该领域内的认可度；②发表文章的主题；③发表文章的类型；④受众；⑤收录情况及影响因子；⑥是否收取版面费；⑦稿件接受率；⑧发表时间等因素。

锁定目标期刊之后，应注册并登录该期刊网站，详细阅读目标期刊的作者指南（guide for authors）。作者指南中通常会说明目标期刊在学术伦理（ethics）、稿件结构（manuscript organization）、文件格式（document format）、发表费用（publication fees）、语言（language）、提交方式（way of submission）等方面的要求。

按目标期刊要求和引导在期刊网站投稿之后，提交的稿件会由一位编辑接收和处理。对于质量较差、原创性不够、不符合期刊定位、选题陈旧、选题已被业内过度探讨或发表的文章，责任编辑可能会在几天甚至几个小时内拒稿（desk rejection）或建议转投（referral），但这也意味着作者可以更快改进以继续投给其他期刊。如果没有直接拒稿或建议转投，编辑会将初稿发给该专业领域的 2~3 位审稿人进行审稿。作者可以在投稿的时候选择双盲（double-blind）或者单盲（single-blind）审稿，有的期刊也允许作者提名审稿人（nominate reviewer）。

审稿过程一般需要 3 个月以上的时间，甚至 1 年以上，这通常取决于稿件进入审稿环节的次数及审稿人的效率。通常情况下每位审稿人都会对稿件提出问题和修改建议，这对于作者来说是一个备受打击却受益匪浅的过程。作者需要冷静面对审稿人的意见，不能有抵触情绪，但也不能在未经考证的情况下全盘接受审稿人的修改意见。作者一定要对应审稿意见逐条回复，对于有必要修改的部分，要在文稿对应的位置认真修改，或给出让审稿人信服的论证，让审稿人看到作者认真严谨的态度。

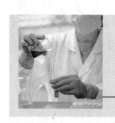

国际期刊通常会要求作者在提交论文的同时附上一封投稿信件（Cover letter）。编辑通常会只阅读投稿信和论文摘要，就决定是否将稿件送审。因此，投稿信的书写质量非常重要，它是作者与编辑直接交流、表达论文重要性、让编辑对本研究感兴趣的机会。

书写投稿信时还应注意：①投稿信篇幅不宜过长；②因为投稿时需要提交摘要，作者在投稿信里不要概括或重复论文摘要；③尽量避免使用专业术语或缩略语，要使用简洁的语言；④避免拼写和语法错误；⑤参照目标期刊所规定的格式和内容要求进行书写。

投稿信通常会涉及表 10-1 中的内容，写作时可以参考表 10-2 中的投稿信模板。

表 10-1　投稿信内容

Address the editor by the name.	称呼编辑姓名
Include your manuscript's title and the name of the journal.	论文初稿标题及目标期刊名称
Provide the author list.	罗列所有作者的姓名
Provide the mailing address, phone number, and email of the corresponding author.	提供通讯作者的地址、电话及邮箱
State the reason for sending the manuscript to the journal rather than others.	说明向该期刊投稿的原因
State the objective, main findings and significance of your study.	阐明本研究的目的、主要研究发现及意义
Confirm the originality of the study.	确认本研究的原创性
State that the manuscript has not been previously published and is not simultaneously submitted elsewhere.	声明论文没有在其他期刊发表过，没有一稿多投
Suggest potential reviewers to include or exclude.	推荐审稿人或要避开的审稿人

(continued)

Declare any conflicts of interest, or confirm there are none.	说明相关利益冲突，或确定没有利益冲突

表 10-2　投稿信模板

Dear ×××（编辑姓名），

　　I'm honored to submit my manuscript entitled "×××（初稿标题）" to be considered for publication in ×××（期刊名称）.

　　A full list of the names of all the coauthors and the contact information of the corresponding author is attached. The coauthors of the manuscript have all approved the manuscript for submission.

　　The article is particularly appropriate for the journal's section dedicated to ×××（所投期刊版块主题）.

　　The research reported in the manuscript I am submitting today was designed to investigate ×××（研究目的）. We found that ×××（研究发现）. Thus, we trust that your readers will benefit from our study as our findings will allow them to understand ×××（研究意义）.

　　I declare that this manuscript is original and has not been published before. It is not currently being considered for publication elsewhere.

　　I believe that the following individuals would be well suited to reviewing my manuscript:

　　Dr. ×××, University of ×××, Professor specializing in ×××: ×××@×××

　　Dr. ×××, University of ×××, Associate Professor specializing in ×××: ×××@×××

　　Dr. ×××, University of ×××, Associate Professor specializing in ×××: ×××@×××

　　To the best of my knowledge, none of the above-suggested persons has any conflict of interest, financial or otherwise.

　　Many thanks for your time and consideration. I look forward to your response.

　　Sincerely,

　　×××

　　AUTHORS:

　　×××

　　AUTHORS' ADDRESSES:

　　×××

　　CORRESPONDENCE AUTHOR:

　　Name: ×××

　　E-mail: ×××

　　Address: ×××

　　Phone: ×××

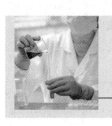

　　在作者提交稿件之后通常会收到拒稿（reject）、大修（major revision）或小修（minor revision）三种回复，很少会有文章在没有经过修改的情况下直接被接受（accept）。当编辑根据审稿人意见要求作者对稿件进行修改（大修或小修）时，这往往意味着作者按照修改意见认真修改是有希望发表文章的。审稿人通常基于以下问题提出修改意见：作者是否明确表达了研究目标、是否清晰阐述了研究方法、研究方法是否具有可复制性、是否清晰描述了所使用的统计分析工具及方法、图表设计是否合理、结果部分是否有充分的数据支撑、是否强调了研究优势及意义、是否说明了研究局限性、稿件结构是否需要改进、语言是否需要润色等。

　　期刊一般都会要求作者基于每条修改意见按照期刊修改格式进行逐条修改。作者提交修改稿的同时，往往还需要提交一封认真书写的回复信（Response letter）来配合修改稿。

　　回复信的作用在于它可以向审稿人和编辑表明你认真积极的修改反馈态度，并可以让他们更直观快速地了解稿件的修改情况。回复信的写作结构是否清晰、回复语气措辞是否恰当等因素都会影响文章是否被编辑和审稿人接纳。回复信通常包含表 10-3 中所罗列的内容及注意事项。

表 10-3　回复信内容及注意事项

Thank the reviewers and editors for their time and comments.	感谢审稿人和编辑付出的时间和给出的修改意见
Address all points raised by the editor and reviewers.	解决编辑和审稿人提出的所有问题
Describe the revisions to your manuscript in your response letter followed by **point-by-point responses** to the comments raised.	在回复信中描述对稿件作出的修改，然后对提出的修改意见逐个回应

(continued)

Perform additional experiments or analyses the reviewers recommend. If you feel that they would not improve your paper, please provide sufficient explanation.	执行审稿人推荐的其他实验或分析。如果你觉得这样并不能改善你的论文，请提供充分的解释
Provide a polite and scientific **rebuttal** to any points or comments you disagree with.	对任何你不赞同的修改意见进行礼貌和科学的反驳
Differentiate between reviewer comments and your responses in your letter, for example, using different fonts.	区分审稿人提出的修改意见和你在信中的回复，例如使用不同字体
In addition to describing the changes in the response letter, show the revisions in the text clearly, either with a different color text, by highlighting the changes, or with **Microsoft Word's Track Changes tool**.	除了在回复信中描述修改内容，还应在稿件中清楚显示修改之处，可以使用不同颜色的文本，突出显示更改内容，或者使用 Microsoft Word 的"修订"工具
Submit the response letter and revised manuscript within the allotted time.	在规定时间内提交回复信和修改后的稿件

表 10-4 的回复信样例中包含了以下内容：①感谢审稿人和编辑对文章给出的修改意见；②给出稿件标题和编号；③表示修改意见对本研究有很大帮助；④描述作者在稿件中如何标记凸显所修改的部分；⑤描述如何区分审稿人提出的修改意见和作者的回复；⑥罗列修改意见，并逐条回应；⑦对不赞同的修改意见进行礼貌和科学的反驳。要注意的是，作者尽量不要轻易反驳编辑和审稿人的意见，除非有足够的理由。

表 10-4　回复信样例

Dear ××× （编辑姓名），

Thank you for the comments on our manuscript entitled "××× （稿件标题）" (ID：×××[稿件编号]). Those comments are very helpful for revising and improving our paper, as well as the important guiding significance to other research. We have studied the comments carefully and made corrections which we hope meet with approval. The main corrections are in the manuscript and the responds to the comments are as follows (the replies are highlighted in bold italics). In the revised manuscript file we highlighted the revisions by using Microsoft Word's Track Changes tool. We also added the corresponding "Author Response" alongside the revised part for you to understand the revised parts easier.

Comment from Reviewer 1: Research questions and objectives are to be clearly stated in a separate section, or explicitly worded toward the end of the Introduction.

Author response: Thank you for pointing this out. We have worded the research objectives explicitly toward the end of the Introduction section.

医学论文英文写作

Comment from Reviewer 2: I think it is better to remove the subheading which reads "Literature review".

Author response: We appreciate your suggestion. However, we think it seems more explicit to set literature review as a separate section to establish a thorough and systematic research context.

Comment from Reviewer 3: The authors mention that "This study only describes statistically significant results." Why is that? Are statistically non-significant results unimportant? Does statistical significance necessarily mean practical significance? It would be meaningful to report all the results in relation to your study objectives regardless of their statistical significance.

Author Response: We agree with you in that we should report all the results in relation to our objective regardless of the statistical significance. We have reported and highlighted the insignificant results related to the objectives in the revision. (See paragraph 3 of the Results section)

Comment from Review 3: Nothing is mentioned about the limitations of this study.

Author response: Thank you for your suggestion. We have revised this part to comment on the limitation of the current study. (See paragraph 4 of the Conclusion section)

Once again, thank you very much for your constructive comments and suggestions which would help us improve the quality of the paper.

Sincerely,
××× (通讯作者姓名)
E-mail: ×××@××× (通讯作者邮箱)

作者撰写回复信时，可以借鉴以下表达：

① 表达感谢。

We are grateful to the reviewers for their positive feedback on our manuscript.

We appreciate the reviewers' recognition of the significance of our research.

Once again, we would like to extend our sincere thanks to the reviewers and editors for their time and valuable feedback.

We are grateful for the opportunity to enhance the quality of our manuscript through this peer review process.

② 概括性地表示进行了修改。

We made the suggested changes to the manuscript as recommended by the reviewers.

The suggested revisions were incorporated into the manuscript to improve clarity.

We carefully considered the reviewers' comments and made substantial revisions to address their concerns.

In response to the reviewers' recommendations, we have conducted additional experiments and analysis, and the results are included in the revised manuscript.

③ 表示赞同。

We agree with you that…

You are right to point out that…

In accordance with the reviewers' comment…

④ 表示不赞同。

While we appreciate the reviewer's perspective, we respectfully disagree with this suggestion for the following reasons…

We understand the concern raised by the reviewer, but our methodology was chosen based on sound scientific principles, as explained in our manuscript.

On balance we prefer to keep our original pattern for the following reason…

⑤ 说明具体的修改。

To address… mentioned by the reviewer, we included … in the manuscript.

We revised the text to provide a clearer explanation of …

We have now changed … into…

We have modified…

More information about…has been provided according to the requirements.

由于审稿人审阅稿件通常都是无偿的，作者书写回复信时应始终采用积极、感激、尊重的语气和态度，尽最大努力高质量地完成所有修改工作。

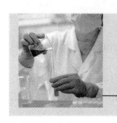

　　论文的审稿和编辑过程可能长达几个月甚至 1 年以上，这取决于期刊审稿周期和论文质量。在选择目标期刊时，作者应该查看期刊网站，了解期刊的发表周期。作者投稿或提交修改稿之后，期刊一般需要 1~2 个月的时间处理稿件并作出决定。

　　如果作者确定自己没有收到任何来自期刊的回复，可以写信向编辑了解稿件目前的进展情况。然而，在联系期刊编辑之前，等待适当的时间是很重要的，因为过于匆忙而频繁的询问可能会让繁忙的编辑产生不悦情绪而影响其对于稿件的决定。

　　如果等待时间过长或者出于特殊原因需要论文尽快发表，作者可以按照期刊要求发送问询信（inquiry letter）。首先，要确定正确的联系人，避免一次给多人发邮件；其次，要用礼貌而尊重的语气；再者，问询信发出之后，作者要保持耐心，尽量避免在等待期间发送多封后续邮件，除非很长时间内没有收到编辑的回复。最后，收到编辑回复后，如果邮件内并没有说明无须回复，作者需要尽快作出回应。

　　询问论文的状态是投稿过程中重要的一步。作者可以参考表 10-5 中的问询信样例掌握其写作方法。

表 10-5　问询信样例

Manuscript Number: ×××（稿件编号）

Dear Mr./Ms. ×××（编辑姓名），

　　Sorry for bothering you. I'm not sure if it is the right time to contact you to inquire about the status of our manuscript titled "×××（稿件标题）", which we submitted to ×××（期刊名称）on ×××（稿件提交日期）.

　　We understand that the peer review process can be time-consuming, and we appreciate the efforts of the reviewers and the editorial team in evaluating our work. However, the status of "Decision in Process" has been lasting for about ×××（稿件提交后至今时长）. I would appreciate it a lot if you could spend some of your time checking and providing an update on the current status of our manuscript.

　　If any additional information or revisions are required, please do not hesitate to inform us. Thank you for your time and understanding.

　　Looking forward to your response.

Sincerely,

×××（通讯作者姓名）

×××（通讯作者联系方式）

附录一
常用医学英语词素

a- ,an-	无，没有
ab-, abs-	离，从，异
ad-	近，向，至
adeno-	腺
-al, -ary	表示…的，与…有关的，像…的
ambi-	双，两，两侧，围绕
amyl-, amylo-	淀粉
ana-	向上，分开
angi-, angio-	血管
ante-	在…之前
anti-	抗，反对
arteri-, arterio-	动脉
-ase	酶
-ate	盐
athero-	脂肪变性，动脉粥样化
arthr-, arthro-	关节
audi-	听，听觉
aur-, auri-, auro-	耳
aut-, auto-	自己，自体，自动
bi-	二，双
bio-	生命，生物
bronch-, bronchi-, broncho-	支气管
carcin-, carcino-	癌

cata-	下，向下
-cele	疝，膨出，肿物
centi-	百分之一
cephal-, cephalo-	头
cervic-, cervico-	颈，宫颈
chir-, chiro-	手
chlor-, chloro-	氯
chol-	胆汁
chrom-, chromat-, chromo-	颜色
chron-, chrono-	时间
-cide	杀
co-, col-, com-, con-, cor-	和，共，相关
crani-, cranio-	颅骨
cyan-, cyano-	深蓝，青紫，绀
cyst-, cysti-, cysto-	膀胱，囊
cyt-, cyto-	细胞
-cyte	细胞
de-	脱离，去掉
deca-	十
deci-	十分之一
dent-, denti-	牙齿
derm-, derma-, dermat-, dermato-,dermo-	皮肤
dis-	不，分离，除去
duo-	二
-ectomy	切除术
encephal-, encephalo-	脑
enter-, entero-	肠
erythr-, erythro-	红色
ex-	外，离，除去，以前的
extra-	外，在外，额外

fibr-, fibro-	纤维
gastr-, gastro-	胃
gluco-	葡萄糖
glycol-	糖
gon-, gono-	种子，精子
granul-, granulo-	粒，颗粒
-graph	描记仪
gyn-, gyne-, gyneco-, gyno-	女性
hector-	一百
hemi-	偏，半，一侧
hepat-, hepatico-, hepato-	肝
hept-, hepta-	七
hist-, histio-, histo-	组织
homeo-	相同
hydr-, hydro-	水，氢
hyper-	超过，过多，高，在⋯之上
hypo-	低，过少，不足，在⋯之下
hyster-, hysteron-	子宫，癔病
-ia, -iasis	病症，情况，病态
-ic	与⋯有关的，产生⋯的，⋯似的
-ics	⋯学，活动，治疗（剂）
-in,-ine	⋯素
in-	不，在⋯内
inter-	间，中间
intra-, intro-	内，内部
-ism	情况，状态，病情
iso-	等，同
-itis	炎症
kilo-	千
lact-, lacti-, lacto-	乳，乳酸

laparo-	腹，腹壁
laryng-, laryngo-	喉
-lepsy	发作
leuk-, leuko-	白色
lip-, lipo-	脂肪，脂类
lith-, litho-	石，结石，钙化石
-logy	…学
lymph-, lympho-	淋巴
lys-, lyso- lysis	溶解，分离
macr-, macro-	大，长，巨
mal-	坏，不良
mamm-, mamma-, mammo-	乳房
mega-	巨大，一百万
melan-, melano-	黑色
men-, meno-	月经
mening-, meningo-	脑膜
ment-, mento-	下巴颏
mes-, meso-	正中，中间，中位
meta-	改变，在…后
-meter	计量器
micr-, micro-	微，细，小
milli-	千分之一
mon-, mono-	单，一
morpho-	形状，形态
my-, myo-, muscul-, musculo-	肌肉
myel-, myelo-	髓，骨髓，脊髓
nas-, naso-	鼻
necr-, necro-	坏死，死亡
neo-	新
nephr-, nephron-	肾

octo-	八
-oid	像…的，类…的
-oma, -omata	瘤
onco-	瘤，肿块
ophthalm-, ophthalmo-	眼
-opia	视力
or-, ori-, oro-	口
-ose	糖
-osis	病，病态
ost-, oste-, osteo-	骨
ovary-, ovario-	卵巢
oxy-	氧，氧化，尖锐
pan-, pant-, panto-	全（部），泛
para-	旁，副，类，拟，异常
path-, patho-, -pathy	病
ped-, pedi-, pedo-	儿童，足
penta-	五
per-	通过，完全
pharmaco-	药，药学
phil-, philo-, -philia	嗜，亲，化学亲和力
-phobia	恐惧症
phon-, phono-	音，声
phos-, phot-, photo-	光
-phrenia	膈，精神
-phylaxis	防御，保护
-plasia	形成，发育，生长
plasma-, plasma-, plasmato-	血浆
-plegia	麻痹，瘫痪
pleur-, pleura-, pleuro-	胸膜，肋膜
-pnea	呼吸

pneum-, pneuma-, pneumat-, pneumato-	肺，呼吸，气体
pod-, podo-	足
poly-	多，多数
post-	后，在…之后
pre-, pro-	先于，在…之前
pseud-, pseudo-	假，伪
psych-, psyche-,psycho-	精神，心理
pyo-	化脓，脓
quadr-, quadri-	四
radio-	放射，辐射，桡骨
re-	再，又
rect-, recto-	直肠
ren-, reno-	肾
retro-	向后，倒退，追溯
rhin-, rhino-	鼻
sarco-	肉，肌
schiz-, schizo-	裂，分裂
scler-, sclera-	硬化，巩膜
-scope	…（检查）镜，观测仪器
-scopy	…镜检查法
semi-	半
sept-, septo-,septi-	七，隔，鼻中隔
sin-, sino-, sinu-	窦
somat-, somato-, somatico-	身体，躯体
staphyl-, staphylo-	葡萄，葡萄状，悬雍垂
-stasis	停滞
steno-	狭窄，狭小
stom-, stoma-, stomat-, stomato-	口，口腔
sub-	在…之下，低于，次于，亚于，副
super-	在…之上，超过，优于

sy-, syl-, sym-, syn-, sys-	相同，共，合
tachy-	快，速，急促
tel-, tele-	远的，远距
tetra-	四
therm-, thermo-	热，温
thorac-, thoracico-, thoraco-	胸，胸廓
thromb-, thrombo-	血小板，血栓
thyr-, thyro-	甲状腺
trache-, trachea-	气管
trans-	经（由），横，贯穿，透过，转移
tri-, tris-	三
-trophy	食物，营养
-tropic	向…的
ultra-	超，超过
uni-	单，一
-uria	尿（症）
uro-	尿，尿道
vas-, vasculo-, vaso-	管，血管
vesic-, vesico-	膀胱，水泡，囊
zo-, zoo-	动物

附录二
常用医学英语词汇

abdomen	*n.* 腹，腹部
abdominal	*adj.* 腹部的
abdominocentesis	*n.* 腹腔穿刺术
abduction	*n.* 外展
abiotic	*adj.* 非生物的，无生命的
abnormality	*n.* 异常，畸形
aborticide	*n.* 堕胎药，堕胎
abortion	*n.* 流产，堕胎，小产
abscess	*n.* 脓肿
absorption	*n.* 吸收
abuse	*n.* 滥用
ache	*n.* 疼痛
acid	*n.* 酸
acidity	*n.* 酸度，酸性
acidosis	*n.* 酸中毒
acne	*n.* 痤疮，粉刺
acquired	*adj.* 后天的，获得的
acrocyanosis	*n.* 手足发绀
acrodermatitis	*n.* 肢端皮炎
acromegaly	*n.* 肢端肥大症
activation	*n.* 激活
acupuncture	*n.* 针灸
acute	*adj.* 急性的

addiction	*n.* 上瘾
adduction	*n.* 内收
adenectomy	*n.* 腺切除术
adenitis	*n.* 腺炎
adenocarcinoma	*n.* 腺癌，恶性腺瘤
adenoma	*n.* 腺瘤
adermia	*n.* 无皮（畸形）
adhesion	*n.* 黏附
adhesive	*adj.* 粘连的
adipose	*adj.* 脂肪的
admission	*n.* 入院
admit	*v.* 住院，为……办理入院手续
adolescence	*n.* 青春期
adrenalin	*n.* 肾上腺素
advanced	*adj.* 晚期的
adverse	*adj.* 不利的，相反的
aerobic	*adj.* 需氧的
aerosol	*n.* 气溶胶
affect	*v.* 感染，（疾病）侵袭
agent	*n.* 药剂
aggravate	*v.* 加重，使恶化
aging	*n.* 老化
agitation	*n.* 激动不安
airway	*n.* 气道
albumin	*n.* 白蛋白
albuminuria	*n.* 蛋白尿
aldosterone	*n.* 醛固酮
alcohol	*n.* 酒精，乙醇
alimentary	*adj.* 食物的，营养的
alkalosis	*n.* 碱中毒

allergen	*n.* 过敏原
allergic	*adj.* 对…过敏的
allergy	*n.* 过敏症
alleviate	*v.* 减轻，缓和
alopecia	*n.* 脱发
alveoli	*n.* 肺泡，齿槽
alveolitis	*n.* 肺泡炎，牙槽炎
amblyopia	*n.* 弱视
ambulance	*n.* 救护车
ameliorate	*v.* 改善，减轻
amenorrhea	*n.* 闭经，无月经，月经不调
amnesia	*n.* 健忘症
amniocentesis	*n.* 羊膜穿刺术
amniography	*n.* 羊水造影术
amnion	*n.* 羊膜
amphiarthrosis	*n.* 微动关节
amputation	*n.* 截肢
amylase	*n.* 淀粉酶
analgesia	*n.* 痛觉缺失
analgesic	*n.* 镇痛剂
	adj. 止痛的，不痛的
anatomy	*n.* 解剖，解剖学
androgen	*n.* 雄激素
anemia	*n.* 贫血，贫血症
anesthesia	*n.* 麻醉，感觉缺乏
anesthesiology	*n.* 麻醉学
anesthetic	*adj.* 麻醉的，感觉缺失的
	n. 麻醉剂
aneurism	*n.* 动脉瘤
angiofibroma	*n.* 血管纤维瘤

angiography	*n.* 血管造影术
angiospasm	*n.* 血管痉挛
angiostenosis	*n.* 血管狭窄
ankle	*n.* 踝关节，踝
anodontia	*n.* 牙缺失
anorexia	*n.* 厌食，神经性厌食症
anoxia	*n.* 缺氧症
antacid	*n.* 抗酸剂
antagonist	*n.* 拮抗剂
antibiotics	*n.* 抗生素
antibody	*n.* 抗体
antidepressant	*n.* 抗抑郁药物
antiemetic	*n.* 止吐剂
antigen	*n.* 抗原
antipsychotic	*n.* 抑制精神病药
antisepsis	*n.* 防腐，消毒，抗菌
antitoxin	*n.* 抗毒素
antiviral	*adj.* 抗病毒的
anti-inflammatory	*adj.* 抗炎的，消炎的
anuria	*n.* 无尿，无尿症
anus	*n.* 肛门
anxiety	*n.* 焦虑
aorta	*n.* 主动脉
aplasia	*n.* 发育不全
apnea	*n.* 窒息，呼吸暂停
apoptosis	*n.* 细胞凋亡
appendectomy	*n.* 阑尾切除术
appendicitis	*n.* 阑尾炎，盲肠炎
appendix	*n.* 阑尾，附录
armpit	*n.* 腋窝

arrest	*n.* 心跳停止，心脏病发作
arrhythmia	*n.* 心律不齐，心律失常
arteriogram	*n.* 动脉搏描记图
arteriosclerosis	*n.* 动脉硬化
artery	*n.* 动脉
arthralgia	*n.* 关节痛
arthritis	*n.* 关节炎
arthrodesis	*n.* 关节固定术
arthrography	*n.* 关节照相术
arthroplasty	*n.* 关节成形术
arthrotomy	*n.* 关节切开术
articulation	*n.* 关节
ascites	*n.* 腹水
asepsis	*n.* 无菌，无菌操作
asexual	*adj.* 无性的，无性生殖的
asphyxia	*n.* 窒息
aspirin	*n.* 阿司匹林（解热镇痛药）
asthma	*n.* 哮喘
asymptomatic	*adj.* 无症状的
atherosclerosis	*n.* 动脉粥样硬化，动脉硬化
atlas	*n.* 寰椎，第一颈椎
atopic	*adj.* 特应性的，异位的
atrium	*n.* 心房
atrophy	*n.* 萎缩
atropine	*n.* 阿托品
audiometer	*n.* 听度计，听力表
audiometry	*n.* 听力测定，听力测验法
audition	*n.* 听觉
auscultation	*n.* 听诊（法）
autism	*n.* 孤独症，自闭症

autoimmunity	*n.* 自身免疫
autopsy	*n.* 尸体剖检
autosome	*n.* 常染色体
axon	*n.* 轴突（神经细胞）
bacillus	*n.* 杆菌
bacteremia	*n.* 菌血症
bacteriology	*n.* 细菌学
benign	*adj.* 良性的
biceps	*n.* 二头肌
bile	*n.* 胆汁
bilirubin	*n.* 胆红素
bioavailability	*n.* 生物利用度，生物药效率
biochemistry	*n.* 生物化学
biofeedback	*n.* 生物反馈
biomedicine	*n.* 生物医学
biopsy	*n.* 活组织检查
biotransformation	*n.* 生物转化
bladder	*n.* 膀胱
blepharitis	*n.* 睑炎
blepharoptosis	*n.* 眼睑下垂
blepharospasm	*n.* 睑痉挛
blocker	*n.* 阻断剂
bout	*n.* （疾病的）发作
bradycardia	*n.* 心动过缓
bradykinesia	*n.* 运动徐缓，动作迟缓
bradypnea	*n.* 呼吸徐缓
brainstem	*n.* 脑干
bronchiectasis	*n.* 支气管扩张
bronchiole	*n.* 细支气管
bronchitis	*n.* 支气管炎

bronchoscopy	*n.* 支气管镜检	
bronchospasm	*n.* 支气管痉挛	
bronchus	*n.* 支气管	
calcification	*n.* 钙化	
calcitonin	*n.* 降钙素	
calcium	*n.* 钙	
calculus	*n.* 结石	
callosum	*n.* 胼胝体	
canal	*n.* 管，道	
cancer	*n.* 癌症，恶性肿瘤	
cancerous	*adj.* 癌症的	
capillary	*n.* 毛细血管	
carbohydrate	*n.* 碳水化合物	
carcinogenesis	*n.* 致癌作用	
carcinoma	*n.* 癌，恶性上皮细胞瘤	
cardiac	*adj.* 心脏的，心脏病的	
cardialgia	*n.* 胃灼痛，心痛	
cardiologist	*n.* 心脏病学家	
cardiology	*n.* 心脏病学	
cardiomegaly	*n.* 心脏肥大	
cardiovascular	*adj.* 心血管的	
carpal	*n.* 腕骨	
cartilage	*n.* 软骨	
catabolism	*n.* 分解代谢	
catheter	*n.* 导管，导尿管	
cavity	*n.* 腔	
cecum	*n.* 盲肠	
cell	*n.* 细胞	
cellular	*adj.* 细胞的	
centesis	*n.* 穿刺术	

cephalic	adj. 头的
cephalometer	n. 头部测量器
cerebellum	n. 小脑
cerebrum	n. 大脑
cervical	adj. 颈的，子宫颈的
cervix	n. 子宫颈，颈部
cesarean	n. 剖宫产手术
chamber	n.（身体或器官内的）室，膛
cheilitis	n. 唇炎
cheiloplasty	n. 唇成形术
chemotherapy	n. 化学疗法
chickenpox	n. 水痘
choana	n. 后鼻孔
cholecyst	n. 胆囊
cholecystectomy	n. 胆囊切除术
cholecystitis	n. 胆囊炎
choledoch	n. 胆总管
cholelith	n. 胆石
cholelithotripsy	n. 碎胆石术
cholera	n. 霍乱
cholesterol	n. 胆固醇
chondrectomy	n. 软骨切除术
chondritis	n. 软骨炎
chondromalacia	n. 软骨软化
chromosome	n. 染色体
chronic	adj. 慢性的
chyme	n. 食糜
cilia	n. 纤毛，睫毛
cirrhosis	n. 硬化，肝硬化
clavicle	n. 锁骨

clinical	*adj.* 临床的，诊所的
clinician	*n.* 临床医生
clone	*vt.* 无性繁殖，复制
cloning	*n.* 克隆
closure	*n.* 闭合，封闭
clot	*n.* 凝块，黏团（尤指血块）
coccus	*n.* 球菌
coccygeal	*adj.* 尾骨的
coccyx	*n.* 尾骨
cochlea	*n.* 耳蜗
colic	*n.* （尤见于婴儿的）腹绞痛
colitis	*n.* 结肠炎
collarbone	*n.* 锁骨
colon	*n.* 结肠
colostomy	*n.* 结肠造口术
colpitis	*n.* 阴道炎
colporrhaphy	*n.* 阴道缝合术
colposcope	*n.* 阴道镜
coma	*n.* 昏迷
complaint	*n.* 疾病
complication	*n.* 并发症
compress	*n.* 敷布
computerized tomography (CT)	*n.* 计算机断层摄影术
concentration	*n.* 浓度
condition	*n.* 状况，病情
condom	*n.* 避孕套
congenital	*adj.* 先天的
congest	*v.* 充血
congestion	*n.* 充血
conjunctiva	*n.* 结膜

conjunctivitis	*n.* 结膜炎
constipation	*n.* 便秘
consultation	*n.* 咨询，会诊
contagious	*adj.* 感染性的
contract	*v.* 收缩
contraction	*n.* 收缩
convolution	*n.* 脑回
convulsion	*n.* 惊厥
cord	*n.* 索状组织，索，带
corectopia	*n.* 瞳孔异位
coreoplasty	*n.* 瞳孔成形术
cornea	*n.* 角膜
corneoiritis	*n.* 角膜虹彩炎
coronary	*adj.* 冠状的
corpse	*n.* 尸体
cortex	*n.* 皮质
corticotropin	*n.* 促肾上腺皮质激素
cortisol	*n.* 皮质醇，氢化可的松
costectomy	*n.* 肋骨切除术
cramp	*n.* 痉挛，绞痛
cranial	*adj.* 颅的，与颅骨有关的
craniectomy	*n.* 颅骨切除术
craniocele	*n.* 脑膨出
craniotomy	*n.* 颅骨切开术
cranium	*n.* 颅
culture	*n.* 培养
cutaneous	*adj.* 皮肤的
cyanosis	*n.* 发绀，青紫
cyclosporine	*n.* 环孢素
cyst	*n.* 囊肿，包囊，膀胱

cystectomy	*n.* 囊切除术
cystitis	*n.* 膀胱炎
cystocele	*n.* 膀胱突出（症）
cystoscope	*n.* 膀胱内部检验镜
cytology	*n.* 细胞学
defecation	*n.* 排便
defect	*n.* 缺陷
deformity	*n.* 畸形
degeneration	*n.* 退化，变性
degenerative	*adj.* （疾病）恶化的，变性的，退化的
dehydration	*n.* 脱水
delivery	*n.* 分娩，递送
dementia	*n.* 痴呆
demerol	*n.* 度冷丁（止痛药）
denervation	*n.* 去神经支配
dendrite	*n.* 树突
dentalgia	*n.* 牙痛
dentin	*n.* 牙质
dentist	*n.* 牙科医生
dentistry	*n.* 牙科学
deoxyribonucleic	*adj.* 脱氧核糖核的
depression	*n.* 沮丧，忧愁，抑郁症
derma	*n.* 真皮，皮肤
dermatitis	*n.* 皮肤炎
dermatologist	*n.* 皮肤科医生
dermatology	*n.* 皮肤医学
dermatomyositis	*n.* 皮肌炎
dermatosis	*n.* 皮肤病
detection	*n.* 检测
deterioration	*n.* 退化，恶化

development	*n.* 发展，发育
diabetes	*n.* 糖尿病，多尿症
diagnosis	*n.* 诊断
dialysis	*n.* 透析
diaphragm	*n.* 隔膜
diarrhea	*n.* 腹泻
diarthrosis	*n.* 动关节
diastole	*n.* 心脏舒张
diencephalon	*n.* 间脑
digestion	*n.* 消化
dilation	*n.* 扩大，膨胀
diphtheria	*n.* 白喉
diplopia	*n.* 复视
disability	*n.* 残疾
discharge	*n.* 出院，（液体、气体等的）排出
dislocation	*n.* 脱臼
disorder	*n.* 障碍，失调，疾病
dispensary	*n.* 配药房
distal	*adj.* 末梢的，末端的
diuresis	*n.* 利尿，多尿
diuretic	*adj.* 利尿的
	n. 利尿剂
diverticulitis	*n.* 憩室炎
diverticulosis	*n.* 憩室病
dizziness	*n.* 眩晕
dominant	*adj.* 显性的
donor	*n.* 供体，供者
dopamine	*n.* 多巴胺
dorsalgia	*n.* 背痛
dorsiflexion	*n.* 背屈

dose	*n.* 剂量
drainage	*n.* 引流
dressing	*n.* （保护伤口的）敷料
dropsy	*n.* 水肿，浮肿
drowsiness	*n.* 睡意，困倦
duct	*n.* 输送管，导管
duodenitis	*n.* 十二指肠炎
duodenostomy	*n.* 十二指肠造口术
duodenotomy	*n.* 十二指肠切开术
duodenum	*n.* 十二指肠
dwarfism	*n.* 侏儒症，矮小
dysentery	*n.* 痢疾
dysfunction	*n.* 功能紊乱，机能障碍
dysmenorrhea	*n.* 痛经
dyspepsia	*n.* 消化不良
dysphagia	*n.* 吞咽困难
dysphasia	*n.* 言语障碍症
dysphonia	*n.* 发声困难
dysplasia	*n.* 发育不良，发育异常
dyspnea	*n.* 呼吸困难
dysthymia	*n.* 心境恶劣，精神抑郁
dystonia	*n.* 肌张力障碍
dystrophy	*n.* 营养障碍，营养失调
dysuria	*n.* 排尿困难
eardrum	*n.* 鼓膜，耳膜
echocardiography	*n.* 超声心动描记术
eczema	*n.* 湿疹
edema	*n.* 水肿
efficacy	*n.* 疗效
egg	*n.* 卵子

elbow	*n.* 肘部
electrocardiogram	*n.* 心电图
electrocardiograph	*n.* 心电图仪
electrocardiography	*n.* 心电描记法
electroconvulsive	*adj.* 电惊厥的，电休克的
electrode	*n.* 电极
electroencephalogram	*n.* 脑电图
electroencephalography	*n.* 脑电描记法
electrolyte	*n.* 电解液，电解质
electromyograph	*n.* 肌电图仪
embolism	*n.* 栓塞
embryo	*n.* 胚胎
embryology	*n.* 胚胎学
emesis	*n.* 呕吐
emetic	*n.* 催吐剂
emphysema	*n.* 气肿，肺气肿
enamel	*n.* 牙釉质
encephalitis	*n.* 脑炎
encephalocele	*n.* 脑膨出
encephaloma	*n.* 脑瘤
encephalon	*n.* 脑
encephalopathy	*n.* 脑病
encephalorrhagia	*n.* 脑出血
endocarditis	*n.* 心内膜炎
endocardium	*n.* 心内膜
endometritis	*n.* 子宫内膜炎
endometrium	*n.* 子宫内膜
endoscope	*n.* 内窥镜，内镜
endoscopy	*n.* 内窥镜检查
enteritis	*n.* 肠炎

enterocele	*n.* 肠疝
enzyme	*n.* 酶
epidemic	*adj.* 流行的，传染性的
epidemiologist	*n.* 流行病学家
epidemiology	*n.* 流行病学，传染病学
epidermis	*n.* 表皮
epiglottis	*n.* 会厌
epilepsy	*n.* 癫痫
episode	*n.* （某疾病的）发作期
epithalamus	*n.* 上丘脑
epithelium	*n.* 上皮细胞
erythroblast	*n.* 有核红细胞
erythrocyte	*n.* 红细胞
erythropoiesis	*n.* 红细胞生成
esophagogastrostomy	*n.* 食管胃吻合术
esophagus	*n.* 食管
estrogen	*n.* 雌激素
etiology	*n.* 病因学
eversion	*n.* 外翻
excision	*n.* 切除
excretion	*n.* 排泄，分泌物
exhalation	*n.* 呼气
exhaustion	*n.* 耗尽，精疲力竭
expiration	*n.* 呼气
extirpation	*n.* 摘除术
extremities	*n.* 四肢
failure	*n.* 衰竭
farsightedness	*n.* 远视
fascia	*n.* 筋膜
fasting	*n.* 禁食

fat	n. 脂肪
fatigue	n. 疲劳
feces	n. 排泄物，粪便
femur	n. 股骨
fertility	n. 生育能力
fertilization	n. 受精
fetus	n. 胎儿
fibrin	n. 纤维蛋白
fibroblast	n. 纤维组织母细胞
fibroma	n. 纤维瘤
fibrosis	n. 纤维化，纤维变性
fibula	n. 腓骨
fistula	n. 瘘管
flatulence	n. 肠胃气胀
flexion	n. 弯曲，屈曲
flexor	n. 屈肌
flu	n. 流感
focus	n. 焦点，病灶
follicle	n. 卵泡，滤泡，毛囊
followup	n. 随访
fracture	n. 断裂，骨折
fungus	n. 真菌，霉菌
gall	n. 胆汁
gallbladder	n. 胆囊
ganglion	n. 神经节
gastralgia	n. 胃痛
gastrectasia	n. 胃胀，胃扩张
gastrectomy	n. 胃切除术
gastritis	n. 胃炎
gastroenteritis	n. 肠胃炎

gastroenterology	*n.* 肠胃病学
gauze	*n.* 纱布
gel	*n.* 凝胶
gene	*n.* 基因
genetics	*n.* 遗传学
geriatrics	*n.* 老年病学，老年病人
geriatrician	*n.* 老年病学专家
gerontology	*n.* 老年医学，老年病学，老人学
gingiva	*n.* 齿龈
gingivectomy	*n.* 龈切除术
gingivitis	*n.* 齿龈炎
girdle	*n.* 肢带骨，围绕物
gland	*n.* 腺
glia	*n.* 胶质，神经胶质
globulin	*n.* 球蛋白
glossalgia	*n.* 舌痛
glossitis	*n.* 舌炎
glottis	*n.* 声门
glucagon	*n.* 胰高血糖素
glucose	*n.* 葡萄糖
glycemia	*n.* 血糖过多
glycosuria	*n.* 葡萄糖尿，糖尿
gonad	*n.* 性腺
gout	*n.* 痛风
gum	*n.* 牙龈
gut	*n.* 肠
gynecologist	*n.* 妇科医生
gynecology	*n.* 妇科学
gyrus	*n.* 脑回
harelip	*n.* 兔唇，唇裂

healing	*n.* 康复
heartburn	*n.* 胃痛，心灼热，心痛，胃灼热
heatstroke	*n.* 中暑
hemangioma	*n.* 血管瘤
hematemesis	*n.* 吐血，呕血
hematologist	*n.* 血液学家
hematology	*n.* 血液学
hematoma	*n.* 血肿
hematuria	*n.* 血尿，血尿症
hemiplegia	*n.* 偏瘫，半身麻痹
hemodialysis	*n.* 血液透析
hemoglobin	*n.* 血红蛋白
hemolysis	*n.* 溶血（现象），血细胞溶解
hemophilia	*n.* 血友病
hemoptysis	*n.* 咯血，咳血
hemorrhage	*n.* 出血
hemorrhoid	*n.* 痔疮
hemostasis	*n.* 止血
hemothorax	*n.* 血胸，胸腔积血
heparin	*n.* 肝素
hepatectomy	*n.* 肝切除术
hepatitis	*n.* 肝炎
hepatomegaly	*n.* 肝（肿）大
herb	*n.* 药草
hereditary	*adj.* 遗传的
hernia	*n.* 疝气，脱肠
herniorrhaphy	*n.* 疝缝手术，疝修补术
hindbrain	*n.* 后脑
histamine	*n.* 组胺
histology	*n.* 组织学

history	n. 病史
hormone	n. 激素
hospice	n. 临终关怀
hospitalization	n. 住院治疗
host	n. 宿主
humerus	n. 肱骨
hydration	n. 水合作用
hydrocephalus	n. 脑积水
hydrophobia	n. 狂犬病，恐水病
hydrothorax	n. 胸膜积水，水胸
hygiene	n. 卫生，卫生学，保健法
hypercapnia	n. 血碳酸过多症
hyperplasia	n. 增生，畸形生长
hyperpnea	n. 呼吸过度
hypertension	n. 高血压
hyperthyroidism	n. 甲状腺功能亢进
hypertrophy	n. 肥大
hypocalcemia	n. 低血钙症，血钙过少
hypoglossal	adj. 舌下的，舌下神经的
hypoplasia	n. 发育不全
hypotension	n. 低血压
hypothalamus	n. 下丘脑
hypothermia	n. 低体温
hypothyroidism	n. 甲状腺功能减退
hypoxemia	n. 低氧血症，血氧不足
hypoxia	n. 低氧，缺氧
hysterectomy	n. 子宫切除
hysterocele	n. 子宫疝，子宫脱垂
hysteromyoma	n. 子宫肌瘤
hysterotomy	n. 子宫切开术

ileum	n. 回肠
ileus	n. 肠梗阻，肠阻塞
imaging	n. 成像，影像学
immunity	n. 免疫力
immunodeficiency	n. 免疫缺陷
immunoglobulin	n. 免疫球蛋白
immunology	n. 免疫学
immunosuppressive	adj. 免疫抑制的
immunotherapy	n. 免疫疗法
impairment	n.（身体机能的）损伤，削弱
implantation	n. 移植，植入，移植
impulse	n. 刺激，（神经）冲动
inborn	adj. 天生的，先天的
incision	n. 切口，切开
indication	n. 迹象
indigestion	n. 消化不良
infarction	n. 梗塞
infection	n. 感染，传染
inflammation	n. 发炎，炎症
inflammatory	adj. 发炎的，炎症性的
influenza	n. 流行性感冒
ingestion	n. 摄取，咽下
inhalation	n. 吸入
inheritance	n. 遗传
inhibition	n. 抑制
inhibitor	n. 抑制剂
injection	n. 注射
innervation	n. 神经分布，神经支配
inpatient	n. 住院部，住院病人
inquiry	n. 探究，调查

insomnia	*n.* 失眠症，失眠
inspection	*n.* 检查，望诊
insulin	*n.* 胰岛素
intake	*n.* 摄入（量）
intercostal	*adj.* 肋间的
intermittent	*adj.* 间歇的
intern	*n.* 实习生，实习医师
interstitial	*adj.* 间质的
intervention	*n.* 介入，干预
intestine	*n.* 肠
intolerance	*n.* 不耐受
intracranial	*adj.* 颅内的
intravascular	*adj.* 血管内的
intussusception	*n.* 肠套叠
invasion	*n.* 入侵，侵袭
iodine	*n.* 碘酒
iris	*n.* 虹膜
iritis	*n.* 虹膜炎
irradiation	*n.* 放射
irreversible	*adj.* 不可逆的
ischemia	*n.* 缺血
islet	*n.* 胰岛
isolation	*n.* 隔离
isotope	*n.* 同位素
itchy	*adj.* 发痒的
jaundice	*n.* 黄疸
jejunum	*n.* 空肠
jel	*n.* 凝胶
joint	*n.* 关节，接缝
keratoplasty	*n.* 角膜移植术

kidney	n. 肾脏
labium	n. 唇
lacrimal	adj. 泪的，泪腺的
lactation	n. 泌乳，哺乳期
lactate	n. 乳酸
lactose	n. 乳糖
laminectomy	n. 椎板切除术
laproscopy	n. 腹腔镜检查
laparotomy	n. 剖腹手术
laryngitis	n. 喉炎
laryngopharynx	n. 咽喉
laryngoscope	n. 检喉镜
larynx	n. 喉，喉头
laxative	n. 泻药
lens	n. 晶〔状〕体
lesion	n. 损害，身体上的伤害，机能障碍
leukemia	n. 白血病
leukocyte	n. 白细胞
ligament	n. 韧带
limb	n. 肢，臂
lining	n.（身体器官内壁的）膜
lipase	n. 脂肪酶
lipid	n. 脂类，油脂
lipoma	n. 脂肪瘤
lipoprotein	n. 脂蛋白
liposarcoma	n. 脂肪肉瘤
lithiasis	n. 结石病
lithogenesis	n. 结石形成
lithotripsy	n. 碎石术
liver	n. 肝脏

lobe	*n.* （脑、肺等的）叶	
local	*adj.* 局部的	
lockjaw	*n.* 破伤风，牙关紧闭症	
loneliness	*n.* 寂寞，孤独	
lumbar	*n.* 腰椎	
lump	*n.* 肿块，瘤	
lung	*n.* 肺	
lymph	*n.* 淋巴	
lymphocyte	*n.* 淋巴细胞	
lysosome	*n.* 溶酶体	
macrophage	*n.* 巨噬细胞	
magnesium	*n.* 镁	
malaise	*n.* 不舒服，心神不安	
malaria	*n.* 疟疾	
malformation	*n.* 畸形，变形	
malfunction	*n.* 功能障碍	
malignant	*adj.* 恶性的	
malnutrition	*n.* 营养失调，营养不良	
mammogram	*n.* 乳房 X 线照片	
mammography	*n.* 乳房 X 线照相术	
mammoplasty	*n.* 乳房成形术	
mandible	*n.* 下颌骨	
marrow	*n.* 髓，骨髓	
mastadenoma	*n.* 乳腺瘤	
mastectomy	*n.* 乳房切除术	
mastication	*n.* 咀嚼	
mastitis	*n.* 乳腺炎	
mastocarcinoma	*n.* 乳癌	
maternity	*n.* 母性，妇产科医院	
maxilla	*n.* 上颌骨	

measles	n. 麻疹
medulla	n. 髓质
melanocarcinoma	n. 黑素癌
melanocyte	n. 黑素细胞
membrane	n. 膜
meninges	n. 脑膜
meningitis	n. 脑膜炎
menopause	n. 更年期
menorrhagia	n. 月经过多
menorrhalgia	n. 痛经
menorrhea	n. 行经
menstruation	n. 月经
mesencephalon	n. 中脑
metabolism	n. 新陈代谢
metacarpal	n. 掌骨
metastasis	n. 转移
metatarsal	n. 跖骨
metrorrhagia	n. 子宫出血，血崩症
microbiology	n. 微生物学
microorganism	n. 微生物
microscope	n. 显微镜
midwife	n. 助产士
migraine	n. 偏头痛
miscarriage	n. 流产
mitochondria	n. 线粒体
model	n. 模型
moderate	adj. 轻度的
molar	n. 臼齿，磨牙
mold	n. 霉菌
mole	n. 痣

molecular	*adj.* 分子的
molecule	*n.* 分子
morbidity	*n.* 发病率
mortal	*adj.* 致死的
mortality	*n.* 死亡数，死亡率
mucosa	*n.* 黏膜
mucus	*n.* 黏液
multiple	*adj.* 多发的
mumps	*n.* 流行性腮腺炎
muscle	*n.* 肌肉
musculoskeletal	*adj.* 肌（与）骨骼的
mutation	*n.* 突变
myasthenia	*n.* 肌无力
mycology	*n.* 真菌学
mycosis	*n.* 霉菌病
myelin	*n.* 髓鞘
myelitis	*n.* 脊髓炎，骨髓炎
myelocele	*n.* 脊髓突出
myelogram	*n.* 脊髓 X 光像
myeloma	*n.* 骨髓瘤
myocarditis	*n.* 心肌炎
myocardium	*n.* 心肌，心肌层
myopia	*n.* 近视
myosclerosis	*n.* 肌硬化症
myositis	*n.* 肌炎，肌肉发炎
myospasm	*n.* 肌痉挛
myotonia	*n.* 肌强直
narcotherapy	*n.* 麻醉疗法
nasal	*adj.* 鼻的
nasogastric	*adj.* 鼻饲的

nasopharynx	n. 鼻咽
nausea	n. 恶心
necrosis	n. 坏死，坏疽
needle	n. 针
negative	adj. 阴性的
neonate	n. 婴儿，（不足四周的）新生儿
neoplasm	n. 赘生物，瘤
nephrectomy	n. 肾切除术
nephritis	n. 肾炎
nephrolith	n. 肾结石
nephrology	n. 肾脏学
nephroptosis	n. 肾下垂
nerve	n. 神经
neuralgia	n. 神经痛
neurasthenia	n. 神经衰弱症
neuritis	n. 神经炎
neurocranium	n. 脑颅，神经颅
neuroglia	n. 神经胶质
neurology	n. 神经学
neuron	n. 神经元
neuropathy	n. 神经病
neurotransmitter	n. 神经递质
nocturia	n. 夜尿症
node	n. 节结，淋巴结
noninvasive	adj. 无创的
nonsteroidal	adj. 非类固醇的
norepinephrine	n. 去甲肾上腺素，降肾上腺素
nostril	n. 鼻孔
nourishment	n. 食物，营养品
nucleus	n. （细胞）核

nursing	*n.* 护理
nutriology	*n.* 营养学
nyctalopia	*n.* 夜盲症
obesity	*n.* 肥大，肥胖
obstetrician	*n.* 产科医师
obstetrics	*n.* 产科学，助产术
occipital	*adj.* 枕骨的
occult	*adj.* （血液）（潜）隐的
oculist	*n.* 眼科医生
oncology	*n.* 肿瘤学
onset	*n.* 发作
oophoritis	*n.* 卵巢炎
ophthalmologist	*n.* 眼科医师
ophthalmology	*n.* 眼科学
ophthalmopathy	*n.* 眼病
ophthalmoplegia	*n.* 眼肌麻痹，眼肌瘫痪
ophthalmoscope	*n.* 检眼镜，眼底镜
opium	*n.* 阿片，麻醉剂
oral	*adj.* 口腔的
orbit	*n.* 眼眶
orchitis	*n.* 睾丸炎
orexia	*n.* 食欲
oropharynx	*n.* 口咽
orthopedics	*n.* 矫形术，矫形外科学
orthopedist	*n.* 整形外科医师
orthopnea	*n.* 端坐呼吸
ossification	*n.* 骨化；成骨
osteoarthritis	*n.* 骨关节炎
osteochondritis	*n.* 骨软骨炎
osteoma	*n.* 骨瘤

osteomalacia	*n.* 骨软化，软骨病	
osteomyelitis	*n.* 骨髓炎	
osteonecrosis	*n.* 骨坏死	
osteopenia	*n.* 骨量减少，骨质缺乏	
osteoporosis	*n.* 骨质疏松症	
osteosclerosis	*n.* 骨硬化	
otitis	*n.* 耳炎	
otorhinolaryngology	*n.* 耳鼻喉科学	
outpatient	*n.* 门诊部，门诊病人	
ovarian	*adj.* 卵巢的	
ovary	*n.* 卵巢	
ovum	*n.* 卵子	
oxygenation	*n.* 氧化，氧合作用	
oxytocin	*n.* 催产素，缩宫素	
pacemaker	*n.* 起搏器	
painkiller	*n.* 止痛药	
palate	*n.* 颚	
palpation	*n.* 触诊	
pancreatectomy	*n.* 胰切除术	
pancreatitis	*n.* 胰腺炎	
pandemic	*adj.*（疾病）在全国（或世界）流行的	
paralysis	*n.* 麻痹，无力	
paraplegia	*n.* 截瘫，半身不遂	
parasitology	*n.* 寄生虫学	
parathormone	*n.* 甲状旁腺素	
patella	*n.* 膝盖骨，髌骨	
pathogen	*n.* 病原体	
pathogenicity	*n.* 致病性，病原性	
pathology	*n.* 病理学	
pediatrician	*n.* 儿科医生	

pediatrics	n. 小儿科，儿科学
pelvic	adj. 骨盆的
pelvis	n. 骨盆
penis	n. 阴茎
pepsin	n. 胃蛋白酶
percussion	n. 叩诊
perforation	n. 穿孔
perfusion	n. 灌注，灌流
pericarditis	n. 心包炎
pericardium	n. 心包，心包膜
peristalsis	n. 蠕动
pertussis	n. 百日咳
phagocytosis	n. 吞噬作用
phalange	n. 指骨，趾骨
pharmacodynamics	n. 药效学
pharmacokinetics	n. 药物（代谢）动力学
pharmacology	n. 药物学，药理学
pharmacy	n. 药房，药剂学
pharyngitis	n. 咽炎
pharynx	n. 咽
phlebitis	n. 静脉炎
phlegm	n. 痰，黏液
phobia	n. 恐惧障碍
phonation	n. 发声
phospholipid	n. 磷脂
physician	n. 医师，内科医师
physiology	n. 生理学
physiotherapist	n. 理疗医师
pituitary	n.（脑）垂体
placebo	n. 安慰剂

placenta	*n.* 胎盘
plaster	*n.* 石膏
platelet	*n.* 血小板
pleura	*n.* 胸膜，肋膜
pleurisy	*n.* 胸膜炎，肋膜炎
pneumococcus	*n.* 肺炎球菌
pneumoconiosis	*n.* 尘肺病
pneumohemothorax	*n.* 气血胸
pneumonia	*n.* 肺炎
pneumothorax	*n.* 气胸
polio	*n.* 小儿麻痹症，脊髓灰质炎
polyp	*n.* 息肉
pons	*n.* 脑桥
porta	*n.* 肝门
positive	*adj.* 阳性的
post-traumatic	*adj.* 受伤后的
practitioner	*n.* 执业医生
precaution	*n.* 预防，预防措施
pregnancy	*n.* 怀孕
prescription	*n.* 药方
prevention	*n.* 预防
primary	*adj.* 初级的，原发的，首要的
proctoscopy	*n.* 直肠镜检查
progesterone	*n.* 黄体酮，孕酮
prognosis	*n.* 预后
progression	*n.* 进展
prolactin	*n.* 催乳激素
prolapse	*n.* （身体器官的）脱垂，下垂
pronation	*n.* 旋前
prostate	*n.* 前列腺

prostatectomy	*n.* 前列腺切除术	
prostatitis	*n.* 前列腺炎	
prosthesis	*n.* 假体	
proteinuria	*n.* 蛋白尿	
protraction	*n.* 前伸	
psoriasis	*n.* 牛皮癣	
psychiatry	*n.* 精神病学	
psychology	*n.* 心理学	
psychosis	*n.* 精神病，精神错乱	
puberty	*n.* 青春期	
pulmonary	*adj.* 肺的	
pulp	*n.* 牙髓	
pulse	*n.* 脉搏	
puncture	*v.* 穿刺	
pupil	*n.* 瞳孔	
pus	*n.* 脓	
pyelitis	*n.* 肾盂肾炎	
pyelonephritis	*n.* 肾盂肾炎	
pylorus	*n.* 幽门	
quadriceps	*n.* 四头肌	
quarantine	*n.* 隔离	
radiation	*n.* 辐射，放射物	
radiography	*n.* 放射线照相术	
radiology	*n.* 放射学	
radiotherapy	*n.* 放射疗法	
rash	*n.* 皮疹	
reagent	*n.* 试剂，反应物	
receptor	*n.* 受体	
recessive	*adj.* 隐性的	
recipient	*n.* 受体，接受者	

recovery	n. 恢复，复原，痊愈
rectitis	n. 直肠炎
rectocele	n. 脱肛
rectocolitis	n. 直肠结肠炎
rectum	n. 直肠
recurrence	n. 复发
referral	n. 转诊病人
reflux	n. 返流
rehabilitation	n. 康复
relaxation	n. 放松，缓和
remedy	n. 疗法
removal	n. 切除
renin	n. 肾素
reproduction	n. 繁殖，生殖
resident	n. 住院医生
respiration	n. 呼吸，呼吸作用
respiratory	adj. 呼吸的
retina	n. 视网膜
retinitis	n. 视网膜炎
rheumatism	n. 风湿病
rheumatoid	adj. 类风湿病的
rhinitis	n. 鼻炎
rhinoplasty	n. 鼻整形术
rhinorrhagia	n. 鼻出血
rhinorrhea	n. 鼻液溢
rickets	n. 佝偻病
rotation	n. 旋转
rubella	n. 风疹
rupture	n. 破裂
sac	n. 囊

sacrum	n. 骶骨
saliva	n. 唾液
salpingectomy	n. 输卵管切除术
sanitation	n. 卫生
sarcoma	n. 肉瘤，恶性间叶肿瘤
scabies	n. 疥疮
scalp	n. 头皮
scalpel	n. 解剖刀，外科手术刀
scanning	n. 扫描
scapula	n. 肩胛，肩胛骨
scar	n. 伤痕
schizophrenia	n. 精神分裂症
sciatica	n. 坐骨神经痛
sclera	n. 巩膜
sclerosis	n. 硬化
screening	n. 筛查
scrotum	n. 阴囊
sebum	n. 皮脂
secretion	n. 分泌，分泌物
sedative	n. 镇静剂，止痛药
seizure	n. 癫痫
semen	n. 精液
sepsis	n. 败血症，脓毒病
sequela	n. 后遗症
serotonin	n. 血清素
serum	n. 血清
severity	n. 严重程度
shingles	n. 带状疱疹
shock	n. 休克
shoulder	n. 肩

sign	*n.* 病征
silicosis	*n.* 硅肺病
sinus	*n.* 窦，静脉窦
sinusitis	*n.* 窦炎
skeleton	*n.* 骨架，骨骼
skull	*n.* 头盖骨
smear	*n.* 涂片
somatostatin	*n.* 生长激素抑制素
somatotropin	*n.* 促生长激素
sore	*adj.* 疼痛的
spasm	*n.* 痉挛，抽搐
specific	*adj.* 特殊的，特定的
specificity	*n.* 特异性
sperm	*n.* 精子
spermatogenesis	*n.* 精子发生，精子形成
sphenoid	*n.* 蝶骨，楔状骨
sphincter	*n.* 括约肌
spine	*n.* 脊柱，脊椎
spleen	*n.* 脾脏
splenectomy	*n.* 脾切除术
splenomegaly	*n.* 脾肿大
sprain	*n.* 扭伤
sputum	*n.* 痰
stapes	*n.* 镫骨
staple	*n.* U 形钉
staphylococcus	*n.* 葡萄球菌
stenosis	*n.* （器官）狭窄
sterility	*n.* 不育，无菌
sternum	*n.* 胸骨
steroid	*n.* 类固醇

stethoscope	*n.* 听诊器
stomachache	*n.* 胃痛
stomatology	*n.* 口腔学，口腔病学
strain	*n.* 菌株
streptococcus	*n.* 链球菌
streptomycin	*n.* 链霉素
stroke	*n.* 中风
subacute	*adj.* 亚急性的
subcutaneous	*adj.* 皮下的
sulcus	*n.* 脑沟
supination	*n.* 旋后运动
suppository	*n.* 栓剂，塞剂，坐药
suppression	*n.* 抑制
surgeon	*n.* 外科医生
surgery	*n.* 外科，外科手术
sympathetic	*n.* 交感神经
synapse	*n.* 突触
synarthrosis	*n.* 不动关节
syndrome	*n.* 综合征
synovitis	*n.* 滑膜炎
syrup	*n.* 糖浆
systole	*n.* 心脏收缩
tachycardia	*n.* 心动过速
tachypnea	*n.* 呼吸急促
tarsal	*n.* 跗骨
taste bud	*n.* 味蕾
temporal	*n.* 颞骨
tendon	*n.* 腱
tendonitis	*n.* 肌腱炎
testis	*n.* 睾丸

testosterone	n. 睾酮
tetanus	n. 破伤风
tetany	n. 手足抽搐，强直
thalamus	n. 丘脑
thermometer	n. 温度计，体温计
thoracocentesis	n. 胸腔穿刺术
thrombocyte	n. 血小板，凝血细胞
thrombophlebitis	n. 血栓性静脉炎
thrombus	n. 血栓
thymus	n. 胸腺
thyroid	n. 甲状腺
thyroidectomy	n. 甲状腺切除术
thyrotropin	n. 促甲状腺素
thyroxine	n. 甲状腺素
tibia	n. 胫骨
tinnitus	n. 耳鸣
tissue	n. 组织
tolerance	n. 耐受性
tomography	n. X 线断层摄影术
tonsil	n. 扁桃体
tonsillitis	n. 扁桃体炎
toxin	n. 毒素
trachea	n. 气管
tracheitis	n. 气管炎
tracheostomy	n. 气管造口术
tracheotomy	n. 气管切开术
trachoma	n. 颗粒性结膜炎，沙眼
transfusion	n. 输血，输液
transmitter	n. 递质
transplantation	n. 移植

trauma	*n.* 创伤
triglyceride	*n.* 甘油三酯
trochlear	*n.* 滑车神经
tuberculosis	*n.* 肺结核，结核病
tumor	*n.* 肿瘤
tympanum	*n.* 鼓膜，耳膜
ulcer	*n.* 溃疡
ulna	*n.* 尺骨
ultrasound	*n.* 超声，超音波
umbilicus	*n.* 脐
uremia	*n.* 尿毒症
ureter	*n.* 输尿管
urethra	*n.* 尿道
urinary	*adj.* 尿的，泌尿的
urination	*n.* 排尿
urine	*n.* 尿
urography	*n.* 泌尿造影术
urologist	*n.* 泌尿科医生
urticaria	*n.* 荨麻疹
uterus	*n.* 子宫
uvula	*n.* 悬雍垂，小舌
vaccination	*n.* 接种疫苗
vagina	*n.* 阴道
vagus	*n.* 迷走神经
valve	*n.* 瓣膜
valvulitis	*n.* 心瓣炎
vein	*n.* 静脉
ventricle	*n.* 心室，脑室
vertebra	*n.* 椎骨，脊椎
villi	*n.* 小肠绒毛

virus	*n.* 病毒
viscera	*n.* 内脏
ward	*n.* 病房
wart	*n.* 疣
wheezing	*n.* 哮鸣音，哮喘
windpipe	*n.* 气管
womb	*n.* 子宫
wound	*n.* 伤口
xeroderma	*n.* 皮肤干燥病
xerophthalmia	*n.* 眼干燥症，眼球干燥症
xerosis	*n.* 干燥病
zoster	*n.* 带状疱疹

附录三
常用医学英语缩写

ADHD	attention deficit hyperactivity disorder	注意缺陷多动障碍
AE	adverse event	不良事件
AIDS	acquired immunodeficiency syndrome	获得性免疫缺陷综合征
ALS	amyotrophic lateral sclerosis	肌萎缩侧索硬化
ARDS	acute respiratory distress syndrome	急性呼吸窘迫综合征
BMI	body mass index	体重指数
BP	blood pressure	血压
CAD	coronary artery disease	冠状动脉疾病
CAT	computerized axial tomography	计算机轴断层摄影术
CBC	complete blood count	全血细胞计数
CHF	congestive heart failure	充血性心力衰竭
CC	chief complaint	主诉
CDC	centers for disease control and prevention	疾病控制和预防中心
CI	confidence interval	置信区间
CNS	central nervous system	中枢神经系统
COPD	chronic obstructive pulmonary disease	慢性阻塞性肺疾病
CPR	cardiopulmonary resuscitation	心肺复苏
CSF	cerebrospinal fluid	脑脊液
CT	computed tomography	计算机体层扫描
DM	diabetes mellitus	糖尿病
DNA	deoxyribonucleic acid	脱氧核糖核酸
ECG	electrocardiogram	心电图
ECHO	echocardiogram	超声心动图

EEG	electroencephalogram	脑电图
EMG	electromyogram	肌电图
ENT	ear, nose and throat	耳鼻喉
FDA	food and drug administration	食品和药物管理局
FSH	follicle stimulating hormone	促卵泡激素
GERD	gastroesophageal reflux disease	胃食管反流病
GI	gastrointestinal	胃肠道
GP	general practitioner	全科医生
HAV	hepatitis A virus	甲型肝炎病毒
HBV	hepatitis B virus	乙型肝炎病毒
HCV	hepatitis C virus	丙型肝炎病毒
HDL	high density lipoprotein	高密度脂蛋白
HGB	hemoglobin	血红蛋白
HIV	human immunodeficiency virus	人类免疫缺陷病毒
HPV	human papilloma virus	人乳头瘤病毒
HR	heart rate	心率
HRT	hormone replacement therapy	激素替代疗法
HTN	hypertension	高血压
IBD	inflammatory bowel disease	炎症性肠病
IBS	irritable bowel syndrome	肠易激综合征
ICU	intensive care unit	重症监护室
IM	intramuscular	肌肉内的
IV	intravenous	静脉内的
LDL	low density lipoprotein	低密度脂蛋白
LMP	last menstrual period	末次月经
LP	lumbar puncture	腰椎穿刺
MI	myocardial infarction	心肌梗死
MRI	magnetic resonance imaging	磁共振成像
MS	multiple sclerosis	多发性硬化症

NMR	nuclear magnetic resonance	核磁共振
NP	nurse practitioner	执业护士
NSAID	non-steroidal anti-inflammatory drug	非甾体抗炎药
OCD	obsessive-compulsive disorder	强迫症
OR	odds ratio	比值比
OS	overall survival	总生存期
PCP	primary care physician	初级保健医生
PE	pulmonary embolism	肺栓塞
PET	positron emission tomography	正电子发射体层成像
PMH	past medical history	既往病史
PMS	premenstrual syndrome	经前期综合征
PTH	parathyroid hormone	甲状旁腺激素
RA	rheumatoid arthritis	类风湿性关节炎
RBC	red blood cell	红细胞
RN	registered nurse	注册护士
RNA	ribonucleic acid	核糖核酸
TB	tuberculosis	结核病
URI	upper respiratory infection	上呼吸道感染
UTI	urinary tract infection	尿路感染
WBC	white blood cell	白细胞

参考文献

[1] Ahlstrom D. How to Publish in Academic Journals: Writing a Strong and Organized Introduction Section [J]. *Journal of Eastern European and Central Asian Research,* 2017, 4 (2).

[2] *Appendix B: Some Common Abbreviations: MedlinePlus.* Medlineplus.gov. https://medlineplus.gov/appendixb.html.

[3] Azer S. A., Dupras D. M., Azer S. Writing for Publication in Medical Education in High Impact Journals [J]. *European Review for Medical and Pharmacological Sciences,* 2014, 18 (19), 2966–2981.

[4] Bahadoran Z., Mirmiran P., Kashfi K., Ghasemi A. The Principles of Biomedical Scientific Writing: Citation [J]. *International Journal of Endocrinology and Metabolism,* 2020, 18 (2), el02622.

[5] Bahadoran Z., Mirmiran P., Kashfi K., Ghasemi A. The Principles of Biomedical Scientific Writing: Abstract and Keywords [J]. *International Journal of Endocrinology and Metabolism,* 2020, 18 (1), el00159.

[6] Beech V. *Research Guides: Citation Styles—APA, MLA, etc.: Home.* libguides. marquette.edu. https://libguides.marquette.edu/citationhelp.

[7] Behzadi P., Gajdács M. Writing a Strong Scientific Paper in Medicine and the Biomedical Sciences: A Checklist and Recommendations for Early Career Researchers [J]. *Biologia Futura*, 2021, 72 (4), 1-13.

[8] Bordage G. Reasons Reviewers Reject and Accept Manuscripts [J]. *Academic Medicine,* 2001, 76 (9), 889–896.

[9] Budgell B. S. *Writing a Biomedical Research Paper: A Guide to Structure and Style* [M]. Tokyo: Springer, 2009.

[10] Cotos E., Huffman S., Link S. A Move/Step Model for Methods Sections:

Demonstrating Rigour and Credibility [J]. *English for Specific Purposes,* 2017, 46, 90–106.

[11] Damme H. V. Twelve Steps to Developing Effective Tables and Figures [J]. *Acta Chirurgica Belgica,* 2007, 107 (3), 237–238.

[12] Foley R., Maweni R., Shirazi S., Jaafar H. *How to Succeed in Medical Research: A Practical Guide* [M]. Hoboken: Wiley-Blackwell, 2021.

[13] Gastel B., Robert A. D. *How to Write and Publish a Scientific Paper* [M]. Cambridge: Cambridge University Press, 2017.

[14] Glasziou P., Irwig L., Bain C., Colditz G. *Systematic Reviews in Health Care* [M]. Cambridge: Cambridge University Press, 2001.

[15] Goodman N. W., Edwards M. B. *Medical Writing* [M]. Cambridge: Cambridge University Press, 2014.

[16] Gosden H. "Why Not Give Us the Full Story?": Functions of Referees' Comments in Peer Reviews of Scientific Research Papers [J]. *Journal of English for Academic Purposes,* 2003, 2 (2), 87–101.

[17] Hilary G. D. *Science Research Writing: For Native and Non-Native Speakers of English (Second Edition)* [M]. New Jersey: World Scientific, 2020.

[18] Hochberg M. E. *An Editor's Guide to Writing and Publishing Science* [M]. New York: Oxford University Press, 2019.

[19] Hyland K. *Hedging in Scientific Research Articles* [M]. Amsterdam: John Benjamins, 1998.

[20] Hyland K. Persuasion and Context: The Pragmatics of Academic Metadiscourse [J]. *Journal of Pragmatics,* 1998, 30 (4), 437–455.

[21] Hyland K. Stance and Engagement: A Model of Interaction in Academic Discourse [J]. *Discourse Studies,* 2005, 7 (2), 173–192.

[22] International Committee of Medical Journal Editors. Uniform Requirements for Manuscripts Submitted to Biomedical Journals: Writing and Editing for Biomedical Publication [J]. *Archives of Medical Research,* 2004, 35 (5), 450–464.

[23] Kambhampati S. B. S., Maini L. Formatting References for Scientific

Manuscripts [J]. *Indian Journal of Orthopaedics,* 2019, 53 (3), 381–383.

[24] Kanoksilapatham B. Rhetorical Structure of Biochemistry Research Articles [J]. *English for Specific Purposes*, 2005, 24 (3), 269–292.

[25] Kwan B. S. C., Chan H., Lam C. Evaluating Prior Scholarship in Literature Reviews of Research Articles: A Comparative Study of Practices in Two Research Paradigms [J]. *English for Specific Purposes,* 2012, 31 (3), 188–201.

[26] Lin L., Evans S. Structural Patterns in Empirical Research Articles: A Cross-Disciplinary Study [J]. *English for Specific Purposes,* 2012, 31 (3), 150–160.

[27] Marabelle A., Le D. T., Ascierto P. A., Di Giacomo A. M., De Jesus-Acosta A., Delord J.P., Geva R., Gottfried M., Penel N., Hansen A. R., Piha-Paul S. A., Doi T., Gao B., Chung H. C., Lopez-Martin J., Bang Y.-J., Frommer R. S.; Shah M., Ghori R., Joe A. K. Efficacy of Pembrolizumab in Patients with Noncolorectal High Microsatellite Instability/Mismatch Repair–Deficient Cancer: Results from the Phase II KEYNOTE-158 Study [J]. *Journal of Clinical Oncology*, 2020, 38 (1), 1–10.

[28] Markovac J., Kleinman M., Englesbe M. J. *Medical and Scientific Publishing: Author, Editor, and Reviewer Perspectives* [M]. London: Academic Press, 2018.

[29] Mazumdar P. Writing an Academic Paper for the Purpose of Publication [J]. *Journal of Evolution of Medical and Dental Sciences,* 2021, 10 (20), 1525–1531.

[30] Morley J. *Academic Phrasebank Enhanced PDF Version.* Academic Phrasebank. https://phrasebankresearch.net/.

[31] Muangsamai P. Analysis of Moves, Rhetorical Patterns and Linguistic Features in New Scientist Articles [J]. *Kasetsart Journal of Social Sciences,* 2018, 39 (2), 236–243.

[32] Mungra P., Webber P. Peer Review Process in Medical Research Publications: Language and Content Comments [J]. *English for Specific Purposes,* 2010, 29 (1), 43–53.

[33] Nicoll L. H., Oermann M. H., Chinn P. L., Conklin J. L., Amarasekara

S., McCarty M. Guidance Provided to Authors on Citing and Formatting References in Nursing Journals [J]. *Journal for Nurses in Professional Development,* 2018, 34 (2), 54–59.

[34] Nwogu K. N. The Medical Research Paper: Structure and Functions [J]. *English for Specific Purposes,* 1997, 16 (2), 119–138.

[35] Paltridge B. Learning to Review Submissions to Peer Reviewed Journals: How Do They Do It? [J]. *International Journal for Researcher Development,* 2013, 4 (1), 6–18.

[36] Paltridge, B. Referees' Comments on Submissions to Peer-Reviewed Journals: When Is a Suggestion Not a Suggestion? [J]. *Studies in Higher Education,* 2013, 40 (1), 106–122.

[37] Patrias K., Wendling D. Citing Medicine: The NLM Style Guide for Authors, Editors, and Publishers [J]. *Morphologia,* 2018, 12 (4), 122–129.

[38] Peacock M. Communicative Moves in the Discussion Section of Research Articles [J]. *System,* 2002, 30 (4), 479–497.

[39] Rennie D. The Contributions of Authors [J]. *JAMA,* 2000, 284 (1), 89.

[40] Salager-Meyer F. Hedges and Textual Communicative Function in Medical English Written Discourse [J]. *English for Specific Purposes,* 1994, 13 (2), 149–170.

[41] Samraj B. Introductions in Research Articles: Variations across Disciplines [J]. *English for Specific Purposes,* 2002, 21 (1), 1–17.

[42] Sepehri M., Hajijalili M., Namaziandost E. Hedges and Boosters in Medical and Engineering Research Articles: A Comparative Corpus-Based Study [J]. *Global Journal of Foreign Language Teaching,* 2019, 9 (4), 215–225.

[43] Shashok K. Content and Communication: How Can Peer Review Provide Helpful Feedback about the Writing? [J]. *BMC Medical Research Methodology,* 2008, 8 (1).

[44] Shoja M. M. *A Guide to the Scientific Career: Virtues, Communication, Research, and Academic Writing* [M]. Hoboken, Wiley Blackwell, 2020.

[45] Smith R. The Rise of Medical English [J]. *BMJ,* 1986, 293 (6562), 1591–

1592.

[46] Stenson J. F., Foltz C., Lendner M., Vaccaro A. R. How to Write an Effective Materials and Methods Section for Clinical Studies [J]. *Clinical Spine Surgery,* 2019, 32 (5), 208–209.

[47] Swales J. M. *Genre Analysis: English in Academic and Research Settings* [M]. Cambridge: Cambridge University Press, 1990.

[48] Swales J. M. *Research Genres: Explorations and Applications* [M]. Cambridge: Cambridge University Press, 2004.

[49] Swales J. M., Feak C. B. *Academic Writing for Graduate Students: Essential Tasks and Skill* [M]. Ann Arbor: The University of Michigan Press, 2012.

[50] Thomas S., Hawes T. P. Reporting Verbs in Medical Journal Articles [J]. *English for Specific Purposes,* 1994, 13 (2), 129–148.

[51] Thompson P. J. How to Choose the Right Journal for Your Manuscript [J]. *Chest,* 2007, 132 (3), 1073–1076.

[52] Tullu M. S. Writing the Title and Abstract for a Research Paper: Being Concise, Precise, and Meticulous Is the Key [J]. *Saudi Journal of Anaesthesia,* 2019, 13 (5), 12–17.

[53] Tullu M. S., Karande S. Writing a Model Research Paper: A Roadmap [J]. *Journal of Postgraduate Medicine,* 2017, 63 (3), 143–146.

[54] Wheatley, D. *Scientific Writing and Publishing* [M]. Cambridge: Cambridge University Press, 2021.

[55] Williams H. C. How to Reply to Referees' Comments When Submitting Manuscripts for Publication [J]. *Journal of the American Academy of Dermatology,* 2004, 51 (1), 79–83.